praise for the happy herbi

THE HAPPY HERBIVORE COOKBOOK

Lindsay offers up some helpful tips and recommendations throughout the book to help make the transition into vegan and vegetarian cooking that much easier.

—HEATHER DALE, FITSUGAR.COM

With flavorful and spice-filled recipes [...] Nixon shows that being a vegan doesn't mean to give up good food.

—THEDAILYMEAL AT FOX NEWS

The Happy Herbivore is a fantastic cookbook for a beginner in the vegan cooking world. Not only are the recipes delicious, but the instructions are easy to read and the ingredients are easy to come by.

—LINDSAY GREENFIELD, MIND BODY GREEN

EVERYDAY HAPPY HERBIVORE

These delicious, plant-based recipes may be a sign of the changing times, but they still embody the spirit of Thanksgiving. Add them to your menu this year and they'll be a part of your holiday stories, memories and traditions for years to come.

—NIL ZACHARIAS, HUFFINGTON POST

All [of Lindsay's] dishes are simple enough for everyday eating, but they also pack enough color and flair for a festive holiday table.

—TARA PARKER POPE, THE NEW YORK TIMES

Her premise is that plant-based cooking doesn't have to be a chore, and that if home cooks creatively use ingredients they already have on hand, they can come up with nutritious meals in 30 minutes or less.

—GRANT BUTLER, THE OREGONIAN

HAPPY HERBIVORE ABROAD

Not all of us can jet off for a warm-weather getaway, but we can all take a trip to the kitchen to whip up meals that take our taste buds on a trip around the globe! Lindsay Nixon ... share[s] low-fat, vegan recipes to help us do just that.

—KARLA WALSH, FITNESS MAGAZINE

Most of [Lindsay's] recipes come together in twenty minutes, making them accessible for busy home cooks.

—LAUREN MIYASHIRO, FOODNETWORK.COM

HAPPY HERBIVORE LIGHT & LEAN

Lindsay Nixon knocks it out of the park with Happy Herbivore Light & Lean. Eat these delicious recipes, start engaging in these low-impact exercises, and watch a health kingdom emerge from within.

—RIP ESSELSTYN, NEW YORK TIMES BESTSELLING AUTHOR OF MY BEEF WITH MEAT

No comment can truly capture the totality of Lindsay's magic in the kitchen! Once again, in *Happy Herbivore Light & Lean*, she creatively proves that plant-based eating is not only delicious but also low-calorie and so satisfying.

Lindsay Nixon's blogs, books, and meal plans have helped many adopt and thrive on a low-fat, whole food eating plan that doesn't lack in flavor or variety.

Lindsay Nixon now is a household name in developing cookbooks that have the kind of recipes...that are healthful, tasty, and easy to prepare. Here's another that you need for your collection.

Lindsay not only provides a wealth of creative plant-based recipes but also gives great tips to help you lose weight, gain energy, and feel fantastic. I invite everyone to read this excellent new book and get started on your journey to health.

HAPPY HERBIVORE HOLIDAYS & GATHERINGS

Lindsay's newest book exceeds all of our expectations for creative holiday meals. Meals you make for your family and friends from *Happy Herbivore Holidays & Gatherings* will speak louder than words about the many reasons to eat healthy foods.

Happy Herbivore Holidays & Gatherings provides you with simple recipes to share the joy of great-tasting, healthy cuisine with your friends and family. It's a go-to resource for those special occasions, or anytime!

Lindsay Nixon and I had similar childhoods in ways that count—we both came from families where food was the focus of every celebration. We have both watched mothers and aunties and grandmothers spend all day in the kitchen preparing for every holiday and preparing every dish with love. Lindsay brings all that love and every joyful memory with her into this, her latest cookbook, *Happy Herbivore Holidays & Gatherings*, and better yet, she does it with delicious, healthy plant-based meals that we can all embrace.

Somehow, Lindsay Nixon has done it again. Her food is healthy, familiar, easy, and delicious. You'll eat this food simply for the joy of eating, but will be bettering your health at the same time. Of all the prescriptions I give to my patients, Lindsay's cookbooks are among the most important.

More books in Lindsay S. Nixon's Happy Herbivore Series

The Happy Herbivore Cookbook
Everyday Happy Herbivore
Happy Herbivore Abroad
Happy Herbivore Light & Lean
Happy Herbivore Holidays & Gatherings

The Happy Herbivore

GUIDE TO

Plant-Based Living

LINDSAY S. NIXON

BenBella Books, Inc.
Dallas, TX

This book is for informational purposes only. It is not intended to serve as a substitute for professional medical advice. The author and publisher specifically disclaim any and all liability arising directly or indirectly from the use of any information contained in this book. A health-care professional should be consulted regarding your specific medical situation.

 BenBella Books, Inc.
10300 N. Central Expressway, Suite #530
Dallas, TX 75231
www.benbellabooks.com
Send feedback to feedback@benbellabooks.com

This book has been updated and expanded from its earlier, e-book only edition.
Printed in the United States of America
10 9 8 7 6 5 4 3 2 1

Library of Congress Cataloging-in-Publication Data:
Nixon, Lindsay S.
  The happy herbivore guide to plant-based living / by Lindsay S. Nixon.
     pages cm
  Includes bibliographical references and index.
  ISBN 978-1-941631-00-3 (paperback)—ISBN 978-1-940363-38-7 (electronic) 1. Vegan cooking.
2. Cooking (Natural foods) I. Title.
  TX837.N5755 2015
  641.5'636—dc23
                    2014040707

Editing by Debbie Harmsen, Shannon Kelly,
   Harrison Flanders, and Kellie Coppola
Copyediting by James Fraleigh
Proofreading by Michael Fedison and
   Kimberly Broderick
Indexing by WordCo Indexing Services
Text design and composition by Kit Sweeney
Some interior design elements by Amy Sly
Printed by Versa Press, Inc.
Cover design by Ty Nowicki and
   Sarah Dombrowsky

Photos on pages 12, 20, 69, 87, 98, 99, 132, 134 (top), 144 (right),
   152 (center), 154, 162 (bottom), 165, 167, 170, 175, 180
   (bottom), 183, 189, and 246 by Natala Constantine
Photo on page 169 by Gabriel Deukmaji
Photos on pages 38, 47, 162 (top), 180 (top), 182, and 271 by Kel
   Elwood Photography
Photos on pages 168, 179 (bottom), and 188 (top) by Ira Mintz
Photos on pages 44, 54, and 161 by Neely Roberts
Photos on pages 31, 68, 127, 129, 149, 187 (bottom), 208, 211, 212,
   216, 221, 237, 244, 273–275, 278, and 279 by Jackie Sobon
Additional photography by Lindsay S. Nixon

Distributed by Perseus Distribution (www.perseusdistribution.com)
To place orders through Perseus Distribution:
Tel: (800) 343-4499
Fax: (800) 351-5073
E-mail: orderentry@perseusbooks.com

Significant discounts for bulk sales are available. Please contact Glenn Yeffeth at glenn@benbellabooks.com or (214) 750-3628.

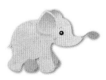

To my parents, Richard and Lenore Shay;
my husband, Scott; my sister, Courtney; my best
friend, Jim; my assistants, Carly, Alison, and
Jamee; all of my Herbies; and every person who
has (or will!) make the plant-based journey on the
highway to health.

contents

a word from lindsay 12

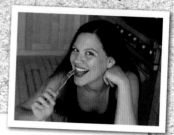

CHAPTER 1
what is a plant-based diet? 19

Plant-Based vs. Vegan 21

The Truth about Plant-Based Nutrition 23

The Dairy Myth 24

The Protein Myth 25

The Grass-Fed Myth 27

The Soy Myth 30

The Oil Myth 31

The "Good Fat" Myth 31

The Fatty Acids (or Fish Oil) Myth 32

The Mediterranean Diet Myth 33

The Vitamin and Mineral Deficiencies Myth 33

The Vitamin B_{12} Myth 34

Plant-Based Food Pyramid 36

CHAPTER 2
why choose a plant-based diet? 39

Health Benefits 40

Chronic Disease 40

Asthma and Seasonal Allergies 43

Hidden Food Allergies and Sensitivities 46

Obesity and Weight Loss 50

Why Are We Obese? 51

The Global Impact of a Plant-Based Diet 55

World Hunger 56

Water Resources 56

Fossil Fuels 57

Other Environmental Factors 60

Human (and Animal) Welfare 61

CHAPTER 3
what to expect 65

Bodily Functions 68

Flatulence 68

Elimination 69

A New (and Improved) Normal 70

Sensitivities and Food Allergies 70

Women and the Plant-Based Diet 71

Pregnancy and Breast-Feeding Nutrition 71

Women and Fertility 75

Contraception 78

Menstruation 80

Menopause 80

Men and the Plant-Based Diet 81

Erectile Dysfunction 83

Prostate Problems 83

Male Pattern Baldness 86

Children and the Plant-Based Diet 86

Athletes and the Plant-Based Diet 94

Pets and the Plant-Based Diet 99

special features

where's the beef? 67

five stages of grief 113

tips for plant-based eating on a budget 116

traveling with my pressure cooker 141

coffeepot pasta 146

food safety 147

two essential camping recipes 148

the mixed-diet hostess 171

hosting potlucks and parties 189

plant-based replacements 194

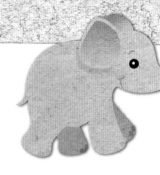

CHAPTER 4
transitioning to a plant-based lifestyle 101
Transition Tips 107
Common Objections 110
  Objection: "Why not 'everything in moderation'?'" 110
  Objection: "Can't I just take a supplement?" 111
  Objection: "Eating healthy is expensive!" 111
  Objection: "I want to have my cake and eat it, too." 112
  Objection: "I'm a picky eater. I don't like [long list of plant foods]. I hate vegetables." 113
  Objection: "But I can't live without [product]!" 117
  Objection: "Cooking takes too much time." 117
  Objection: "We all have to die of something, right?" 118
  Objection: "I don't have willpower." 118
Commercial Substitutes 120
  Plant-Based Commercial Substitutes (Happy Herbivore-Approved Brands) 120
  Vegan (Not Plant-Based) Substitutes: Meat, Cheese, Ice Cream, and More 122
Minimalist Meals 127

CHAPTER 5
plant-based life on-the-go 131
Eating Out 132
  Finding Options 133
  Veg-Friendly Cuisines 134
  Finding Healthy Options—Anywhere 136
Traveling 140
  Plant-Based Travel Foods—What to Pack 141
  Supermarkets and Fruit Stands 144
  Best Bets at Roadside Restaurant Chains 145
  Websites and Apps 145
  Hotels (and Dorms) 146
  Camping and Backpacking 146
  Things to Grill 148
  Vegan Travel Emergency Kit 149

CHAPTER 6
challenges 153
Food Addictions 154
  Breaking Food Addictions 155
  A Note about Cravings 160
  Tasteless Taste Buds 161
Negativity 162
Social Situations 167
  The "Don't Worry about Me" Approach 167
  Dinner Invites 168
  Weddings and Other Catered Events 169
  Kids' Parties 170
  "But I Made This for You!" (Politely Declining Food) 170
  People-Pleasing Pitfalls (and Standing Your Ground) 173
Avoiding Temptation 174
Being "Selfish" 175
Mixed Households 175
Combatting Anecdotal Evidence 178

CHAPTER 7
getting family and friends on board (lead by example) 181
Tailor Your Message So It's Heard 183
Feed Them (the Ultimate Persuasion) 187

CHAPTER 8
cooking, baking, and dealing with allergies 193

Making Substitutions and Adaptations in
Recipes 194

Allergies and Allergy-Free Cooking 196

Soy Alternatives 196
Nut Alternatives 197
Legume (Beans and Lentils) Alternatives 197
Wheat and Gluten Alternatives 198
Corn Alternatives 198
Alternatives for Other Foods 199

Plant-Based Baking 199

Replacing Eggs 200
Replacing Fat (Butter, Margarine,
Shortening, and Oil) 201
Whole-Wheat Flours 202
Gluten-Free Baking 203
Sugar and Sweeteners 203
Cocoa 204
White Chocolate 205
Chocolate Chips 205
Carob 205
Milk 205

CHAPTER 9
troubleshooting: failure to thrive 209

Issue: Not Losing Weight 210
Issue: Feeling Tired and Irritable 211

CHAPTER 10
getting started on your plant-based journey 213

Make a Commitment 214
Just Begin 214
Shopping List 215

Breads and Dry Goods 215
Canned Goods 215
Condiments and Dressings 215
Soy and Nondairy 215
Fresh Produce 215
Freezer 217
Pantry 217
Spices and Dry Herbs 218
Baking 218
Gluten-Free Substitutes 218
Soy-Free Substitutes 218

CHAPTER 11
recipes 219

One-Pot Recipes 221

Bean Soup 222
"Beef" and Broccoli 223
Belize Bean Quesadillas 224
Butternut and Pea Curry 226
Caribbean Ragout 227
"Cheater" Tofu Lettuce Wraps 228
Indian Lentils & Cabbage 229
Lemon Takeout Chickpeas 230
Mexican Quinoa 231
Moroccan Carrot Soup 232
Moroccan Chickpeas 233
Mushroom & Potato Soup 234
Pozole 235
Southwestern Loaf 236

Do-It-Yourself Recipes for
Plant-Based Condiments, Broths,
and Sauces 237

No-Beef Broth 238
No-Chicken Broth 238
AJ's Vegan Parmesan 239
Vegan Mayo 239
Vegan Worcestershire Sauce 240
Golden Dressing 241
Creamy Cajun Mustard 242
Vegan Sour Cream 242
Everyday Mushroom Gravy 243
Ketchup 244
"Honey" Mustard 245
Quick Queso Sauce 245

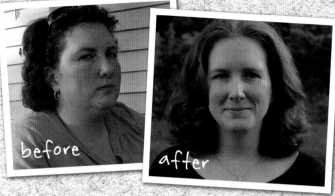

before

after

see beth's full transformation p. 76

APPENDIX

learn more about plant-based living 247

Resources 248

   Animal Welfare 248

   The Environment 249

   Fitness and Athletics 250

   Food Addiction 251

   Health 251

   For Kids 253

   Meat and Masculinity 254

   Parenting 254

   Pregnancy 255

   Religion and Politics 256

Notes 257

About the Author 267

Index 268

testimonials

LINDSAY: my journey on the plant-based highway to health 14

DAVID: once immobile & an addict, now a plant-based bodybuilder 28

CHRIS: finally loving himself thanks to a plant-based diet 37

RUSS: lost 100 pounds on a plant-based diet 58

ELONDRA: college student spreading the plant-based diet on campus 63

BETH: cured from pcos & infertility 76

BRIAN: plant-strong cancer survivor 84

MICHELLE: remarkable changes in kids on a plant-based lifestyle 88

AUBREY: plant-based high school track star 92

SHELDON: retired police officer & plant-based karate champion 96

CAM: eleven-time national champion plant-based boxer 100

MY PARENTS: our daughter talked us into going plant-based and we love it 104

ROBIN: lost more than 200 pounds 114

SALLY: late-stage ovarian cancer survivor 119

AARON: plant-based firefighter 138

TEBBEN: plant-based soldier 150

AMI: former low-carber and ex-cheese addict 158

MICHELLE: overcame an eating disorder 163

JEREMY: plant-proud dad raising a plant-based family 184

KIM: getting the family plant-based 190

GINA: lost more than 100 pounds by switching from "vegan" to plant-based 206

a word from lindsay

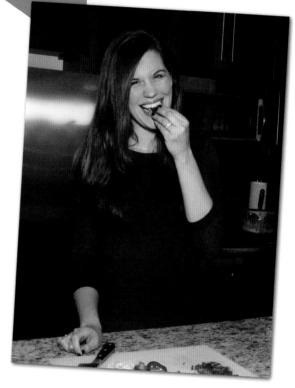

After writing five cookbooks, I looked around to see what I'd left uncovered. I'd tackled comfort foods with *The Happy Herbivore Cookbook*, fast "weeknight" recipes with *Everyday Happy Herbivore*, international recipes with *Happy Herbivore Abroad*, low-calorie recipes (complete with workout plans) in *Happy Herbivore Light & Lean*, plus "fancy pants" holidays, party, and potluck recipes for a myriad of occasions in *Happy Herbivore Holidays & Gatherings*. What was left?

The answer finally came to me, and it couldn't have been more obvious. Day in and day out my fans (called "Herbies") were sending me dozens of questions via e-mail, Twitter, Facebook, my website (happyherbivore.com), and so on. I kept hearing the same questions over and over, and couldn't figure out why. Then it hit me. My cookbooks weren't answering the most basic question: how to live the happy herbivore lifestyle I was encouraging.

Sure, I'd created recipes for how to cook and eat healthy at home, but this isn't a diet—it's a *lifestyle*. Being a happy herbivore and following a plant-based diet extends far beyond what you're cooking next.

What do you do in social situations outside of the home, for example? Or at restaurants? Potlucks? Weddings? When you're camping? What about traveling and vacation? How do you deal with negativity and naysayers? When and how do you talk to your family and friends about your new way of life? And what dishes can you make that even your most skeptical and carnivorous friends will enjoy?

These are the topics of the most frequently asked questions I receive, and now it made sense to me why. I'd taught you how to cook but not how to *live*.

So with this book I have tackled these topics and created a "Herbie handbook"—a practical guide to transforming your life through plant-based eating. From travel resources to unmentionables, I cover every question you'll ever have—and some you'd never have thought of! I also debunk common myths and objections about the vegan lifestyle and plant-based diet. Think of this book as your plant-based bestie, doling out practical advice for *every* situation.

But this book is far more than a multi-page FAQ! You'll also find shopping lists (including lists of specific brands to buy), transition tips, talking points, easy meal strategies (including more than a dozen one-pot recipes!), pictures demonstrating the plant-based lifestyle, and real-life stories from people just like you who jumped on the plant-based highway to health and changed their life in unbelievable ways.

This book is your light (not too science-y!), well-rounded approach to the who, what, how, and why of the plant-based diet. Let's start transforming your life today!

Viva herbivore!

MY JOURNEY ON THE PLANT-BASED HIGHWAY TO HEALTH

As a young child I had a natural intuition toward health. I didn't like meat or cheese (my mom famously told stories about how I'd rip the cheese off pizza and just eat the dough). I also loved fruit and raw vegetables. I still remember once overhearing my mom brag to our relatives, "My Lindsay loves fruits and vegetables. She eats so many vegetables!" She would also gloat about how I didn't care much for candy and that she often had to throw away the candy I collected on Halloween or Easter.

I also deeply loved animals, so when I put it together that hamburgers came from cows and chicken nuggets didn't grow on trees, it wasn't a surprise to my parents that I declared myself a vegetarian.

My parents were mostly supportive, except that they'd occasionally feed me meat and tell me it was soy or vegetarian. (My mom insists I can't still tell this story since she is now plant-based, but I think it paints a good picture. Though when I first figured it out, I held a grudge for several years!)

Yet even though I was a vegetarian, I was a chubby, awkward-looking kid. I can remember my pediatrician telling my eight-year-old self to lay off the mashed potatoes because I "had too much baby fat." I also remember an adult at a pool party pointing out my fat rolls when I was sitting down in a two-piece bathing suit. (I'm thirty-three now and still look down anytime I sit in a bikini.)

The problem wasn't that I was a vegetarian but that I lived on processed foods. Eggos, Toaster Strudels, sugary cereals, Lunchables, and Little Debbies were all the rage when I was growing up. (I also remember my mom once bragging to my aunt that I ate two bowls of cereal for her each morning. That particular cereal was chocolate flavored with marshmallows. Was my affinity for it all that surprising?)

My mom, like a lot of other parents then—and now—had no idea these "convenience" foods were unhealthy. We ate them happily, thinking we were making good choices as a family. After all, that's what their marketing told us!

We also rarely ate out. Restaurants were reserved for special occasions and fast food was all but nonexistent in our diets, especially after I declared myself a vegetarian—there was nothing for me at restaurants to eat (until I discovered bean burritos at Taco Bell in my teens).

Because I was a vegetarian who didn't eat cheese, and I didn't care much for eggs, either, my pediatrician insisted I drink a lot of milk, which my parents made sure I did. Perhaps it's no surprise, then, that I started experiencing migraines when I was eight years old. I had it all: sensitivity to light and sound, severe vomiting, extreme changes in temperature, and a fierce hammering pain behind one eye.

Initially my pediatrician refused to believe I even had migraines given my young age, but eventually I was diagnosed, sent to specialists, and put on varying amounts of pills—none of which worked. Meanwhile I was miserable and often missed sleepovers and birthday parties because I was too busy having a migraine. I also remember my parents crying outside the bathroom door, beside themselves that there was nothing they could do to help me.

As I grew older, I became somewhat slender, though I was never as thin or lean as my girlfriends. I would secretly curse their perfect bodies and wonder, why them and not me? I was also very insecure, but masked it in unhealthy ways.

Eventually I fell out of my vegetarian ways in my late teens from peer and familial pressure, and my health started to worsen immediately. My crippling migraines came with greater frequency. I also developed painful, embarrassing acne and started gaining weight rapidly. My doctor chalked it up to puberty.

In college I lived a busy life—work, class, extracurricular activities, boyfriends—and between my hectic schedule and meager

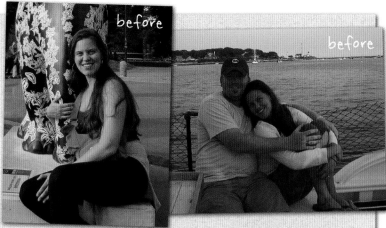
before

before

bank account, I missed meals rather often, though always unintentionally. I slimmed down noticeably early on in college and loved all the attention my new body was getting. For the first time in my life, my friends were jealous of *me*.

I also made friends with other girls who were eager to lose weight, and we would constantly talk about what was healthy, try a new diet together, and exercise when we could at the college gym. With their help, I stayed slim, though not in the healthiest manner.

This continued until my senior year when I met my now husband. A few weeks after we started dating, Scott made a passing comment that when we first went out, he thought I was anorexic and didn't eat. I was mortified. I hadn't ordered much food on our first (or second, or third!) date because I was so nervous and I felt bad that he—someone who was also struggling financially—was graciously paying for my meals. But then I became worried he wouldn't like me because I'd been peckish, and I already liked him so much. So I made a point to eat when I was around him and sort of let loose. I wasn't binging or gorging myself, I was just eating whatever I wanted without pausing to figure out what the healthiest option was, as I used to. If I gained weight, I told myself it wouldn't matter, Scott would love me anyway.

By the time our first anniversary rolled around, both of us were the chubbiest we'd ever been in our entire lives. What's the saying? We were fat and happy.

Scott and I met in January, and by the following fall, I can distinctly remember pulling my winter clothes out and being baffled—truly baffled—why none of them fit. I kept trying them on and wondering what the problem was. *How did all my clothes shrink in the closet? I just wore them eight months ago!* Never did the thought occur to me that I had put on substantial weight. No, no. I was the same. I continued to live in denial until a serious health scare changed everything.

Just as I had been in college, in law school I was busy, juggling a full-time job, classes, and my long-distance boyfriend. I knew I needed to go to the doctor for a regular exam, but I just couldn't find the time. Besides, I was in my early twenties and healthy. *What was the big rush? I wasn't dying!*

Eventually I found the time to go (truthfully, I'd run out of migraine pills and knew I couldn't get more without a new prescription). When the exam was over, I knew something was wrong. My doctor's expression said it all.

My cervix had visitors: precancerous cells and a lot of them. I was shocked. How could I face cancer at such a young age when my whole life was ahead of me? Thankfully it was detected early enough that I could have the cells removed in an outpatient procedure without much disturbance to my life, but the whole experience rattled me. That was my wake-up call.

I started making changes. I joined a gym and started cooking meals at home rather than eating out all the time. Between my newfound exercising and dieting, I was able to slim down a good bit in time for my

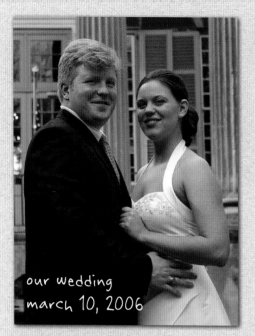

our wedding
march 10, 2006

the plight of farm animals and the ecological consequences of animal products, so on a trip to San Francisco—a town known for being vegan-friendly—I gave it a whirl.

Feeling better than ever, I decided to stick with my new diet when I returned home to Boston, but I was worried about my health— *where would I get my protein and calcium*, I wondered. I read *The China Study* and *Skinny Bitch*, two books that solidified my decision to permanently adopt a vegan diet.

Initially my diet was pretty limited, if not unhealthy: French fries, Boca burgers, PB&J, and pasta with oil was the norm, but the more I learned, and the more I read, the more changes I made. Eventually, I migrated to a 100 percent plant-based diet, eliminating all processed foods. I also removed all added fats and all oils after reading *The McDougall Program*.

My world changed. I lost weight quickly and effortlessly. I also started sleeping better. My acne went away and so did the stomach issues that I thought were "normal." My migraines were all but nonexistent. I also had so much energy that ten months after adopting my new diet, I ran a marathon even though I had been too out of shape to walk a 5K the year before. I started snowboarding and mountain biking—two sports that previously seemed so extreme and beyond my reach.

wedding, though I still wasn't happy with my body.

I then started reading more books on health and nutrition, and before long I found myself migrating back to the vegetarian diet of my childhood. I didn't tell my husband about my dietary change right away. After a few weeks my good friend Stephanie noticed I wasn't eating meat and asked me about it. She then subsequently asked my husband what he thought about his wife going vegetarian (unaware I hadn't told him!) and the proverbial cat was out of the bag.

Luckily, Scott was supportive, though he was intensely firm he would not join me in this new endeavor. We found our middle ground, and slowly but surely I started feeling better and losing weight as a vegetarian.

About a year later I went vegan as an experiment. I'd heard that a vegan diet was great for weight loss and I still had weight to lose. I'd also heard going vegan could clear up your skin, and after a decade of embarrassing acne, I was willing to try anything. There were other motivations as well. I'd become increasingly more aware of

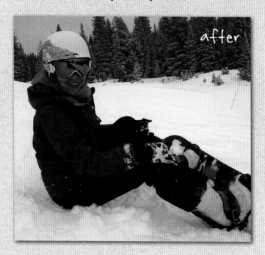

after

Those around me took notice. Friends asked my secret. Strangers asked how I got my glow or my long, shiny hair. It was like that time in college all over again, except this time I'd achieved my healthy appearance in a wholesome way.

Eventually my husband hopped on the plant-based highway to health with me. One day he slipped into conversation at dinner that he had been vegetarian for thirty days. I nearly fell over. Another year or so later he was finally off cheese and 100 percent plant-based. (I may have pushed him to go the extra mile, but he loves being plant-based now.)

My husband's long and embarrassing history with irritable bowel syndrome ended immediately. He was also cured of his eczema, and like me, ran his first marathon as a vegan. Running a marathon was something he never thought he'd be able to do.

Our story doesn't end there, though. After Scott lost over 40 pounds and I lost

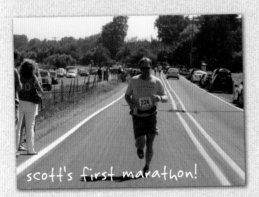
scott's first marathon!

35 pounds or so, and we'd maintained those losses for a while, we started slipping on our plant perfection. We were always vegan, but we started being less strict. We ate vegan junk foods "once in a while" and dabbled in the new vegan commercial substitutes that were hitting the market—vegan cheeses and such that weren't available when we first transitioned.

Although I knew these weren't health foods, I would talk myself into it. Typically I would see a skinny friend eating absolute junk and think, *Well, if they can eat THAT*

and stay slim, surely this pint of vegan coconut ice cream can't ruin me! (Scott's kryptonite was beer, faux meats, vegan pizza, and French fries.)

For the next few years I gained (and lost) the same 10 pounds. My husband, unfortunately, slowly gained back half the weight he'd originally lost. When my clothes felt snug, I would go back to my strict diet. Once I lost the weight again, and I would feel that false sense of security, I would predictably start slipping on my nutritional excellence. Scott just kept gaining.

We both started letting in all those old excuses and justifications we'd used so many years ago that had made us 40-plus pounds overweight: "You only live once." "I'll be perfect on Monday." "I'll go to the gym." "Everything in moderation."

Then I started writing *Happy Herbivore Light & Lean*. I knew a fitness shoot was inevitable, and so I decided to finally get my act together. I was fed up with the 10-pound circuit. I was tired of gaining and losing the same 10 pounds. I committed to my health. No more eating vegan junk foods here

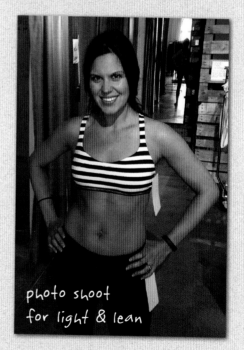
photo shoot
for light & lean

and there. No more eating out two to three times a week and not worrying if it's healthy so long as it's "vegan."

I started following my 7-Day Meal Plans (http://www. getmealplans.com) strictly, and within weeks the 10 pounds had melted off one more time. I was feeling and looking great! Then I lost 3 more pounds, bringing me back to my high school weight. I couldn't believe it! Then I lost more.

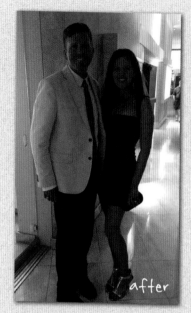

after

It's been over two years now and I've kept off those 10 pounds—a real testament to myself that moderation is just a lie we tell ourselves (see p. 110 for more information). My husband also lost all the weight he'd gained back, plus lost another 25 pounds, bringing his total loss to over 65 pounds! As of this writing he is now the

trimmest and most fit he's ever been in his entire life. More importantly, we don't just look good—we feel amazing.

Since our new "strict" adherence, there have only been a handful of times where we caved and had vegan junk food, and every time it was not worth it. Not only did it not taste as good as we expected or remembered; we found ourselves feeling gross, and more often than not, with stomach pain or gas.

We don't feel deprived by our whole food diet. If anything, eating those nasty foods deprived us of feeling incredible.

I know temptation is hard—you don't have to convince me! There's a reason I don't keep peanut butter and dark chocolate in the house anymore, but it's true: Nothing tastes as good as healthy feels. And more importantly, there is a certain freedom in knowing you can always make a healthy, whole food, plant-based option of whatever you're craving. You are worth it. Your health is worth it. The brownie is NOT worth it!

Coming all the way back to where I started: My poor health came from an assumption—misbelief from misguided propaganda that what I was doing was right and healthy. It was a real education and personal experiment that saved me and my family: my parents, my husband, and my sister, who you will read about in this book. Most importantly, it can save you, too.

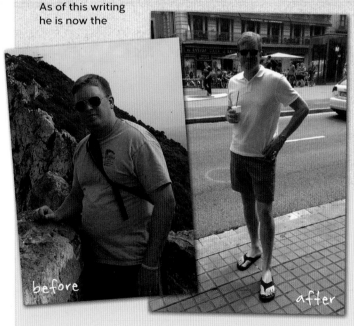

before

after

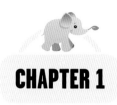

what is a plant-based diet?

"We must get away from the 'diet'
mentality that promotes heroic and unsustainable
spurts of healthy eating. Instead of 'dieting'
we must change our lifestyle to include a diet
that promotes health."

—DR. T. COLIN CAMPBELL, AUTHOR OF *THE CHINA STUDY*—

I loathe the word "diet." It reminds me of all those fad weight-loss schemes that never work, but that restrictive connotation is just the *verb* definition of the word. The *noun* definition of diet embraces *abundance*. "Diet" as a noun represents the array of food a person, animal, or community habitually eats, and that's *exactly* what I'm referring to when I say "plant-based diet" because a plant-based diet isn't a diet at all—it's a *lifestyle*! (A lifestyle that happens to involve a food philosophy ... so let's talk about that first!)

As the name suggests, a plant-based diet is focused around plant foods—fruits, vegetables, legumes, grains, nuts, and seeds—and zero animal products. That means no meat, fish, butter, milk, eggs, cheese, gelatin, or other animal by-products.

Due to the lack of animal products, some people assume plant-based is the same thing as vegan or vegetarian, but that's not necessarily true. Depending on the context, the difference between the two may be subtle or vast.

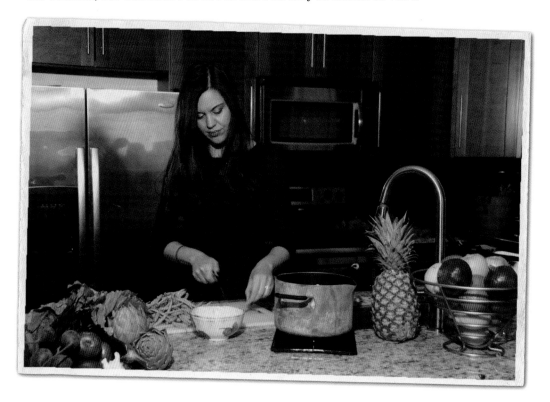

plant-based vs. vegan

Just like the word "diet" means something different when used as a noun versus a verb, the word "vegan" also varies in meaning depending on which part of speech it represents. People who are vegans (noun) not only eschew animal products on their plates but also in their entire lives.

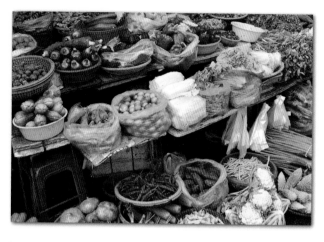

For example, vegans don't wear leather, fur, wool, or silk, or use products tested on animals, due to their ethical beliefs. For this reason, a person who follows a plant-based diet is not necessarily a vegan.

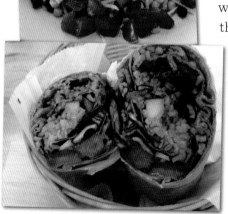

On the other hand, when using the term "vegan" as an adjective to describe *some thing* rather than *someone*, I think of it as meaning there is an absence of animal products.

Meanwhile, "plant-based" is used to describe something that is not only free of animal ingredients, but also made from only whole, unprocessed plant foods. This means that a plant-based meal would qualify as a vegan meal, but a food that is vegan may not be plant-based. For example, potato chips, candy, soda pop, soy cheese, and Oreos are vegan—they contain no animal-related products—but they are not considered plant-based because they are not made only from whole, unprocessed plant foods. *See the difference?*

Here's a little quiz to see if you've got it all straight.

True or False

T F

○ ○ 1. Gelatin comes from the collagen of animals.

○ ○ 2. Oreos are a plant-based food.

○ ○ 3. Soy products are vegan.

○ ○ 4. Someone who follows a plant-based diet might not necessarily shun leather.

○ ○ 5. Honey is both vegan and plant-based.

○ ○ 6. Homemade bean burgers are plant-based.

○ ○ 7. Whey is a milk by-product.

○ ○ 8. Peanut butter is not vegan.

○ ○ 9. The plant-based diet is limited to raw foods.

○ ○ 10. Vegetarians eat eggs and milk but vegans do not.

For the answers, turn this page upside down.

ANSWERS: 1.True 2.False 3.True 4.True 5.False 6.True 7.True 8.True 9.False 10.True

EXPLANATIONS: 2. Oreos don't contain meat, milk, eggs, or other animal by-products, so they are vegan, but because Oreos are a processed food, they are not plant-based. **5.** Some vegans eschew honey (since bees are animals); others do not. **8.** Peanut butter is usually only ground nuts plus salt, sugar, and oil, making it completely vegan. Natural peanut butters that have no added oil and limited amounts of sugar and salt are plant-based. **9.** You can eat raw foods on a plant-based diet, but you're not limited to raw foods. Cooked plant foods like beans, grains, and vegetables are included.

A VEGAN VS. A PLANT-BASED EATER

VEGAN	PLANT-BASED EATER
Eats no animal meat or animal by-products	Eats no animal meat or animal by-products
Wears no clothing made from animals	Eats only whole, unprocessed plant-based foods

the truth about plant-based nutrition

In *The Pleasure Trap*, Drs. Douglas J. Lisle and Alan Goldhamer write, "We are designed by nature to consume the majority of our calories from plants. On this point, there is little dispute among dietary paleontologists. Fruits, vegetables, whole grains, beans, nuts, and seeds have been the dominant source of calories for our species."[1]

Why, then, is our modern diet so different?

Unfortunately, political and financial interests have routinely been put ahead of our health interests.

For example, in 2000, the Physicians Committee for Responsible Medicine won a lawsuit against the U.S. Department of Agriculture (USDA) for unfairly promoting the special interests of the meat and dairy industries through its official dietary guidelines (known then as the Food Guide Pyramid). It was revealed that six of the eleven members of the USDA committee assigned to create the guidelines had financial ties to meat, dairy, and egg interests. (Prior to this lawsuit, the USDA had refused to disclose such blatant conflicts of interest.)

Since numerous books discussing food politics already exist, I won't delve too deeply here except to say that special interests with deep pockets (and clever marketing masked as information) have led us to believe we *need* meat, milk, eggs, and other animal products to be healthy, but that couldn't be further from the truth.

Have you heard any (or all) of the following?

"Where do you get your protein?"

"Without milk, won't all your bones break?"

"Can you get all of the vitamins and minerals from plants that you get from meat and dairy?"

These questions—the result of all that misguided propaganda—are ones you'll likely hear from friends and family once you adopt a plant-based lifestyle. If you're new to plant-based eating, you may be asking these questions yourself.

As with food politics, many books go into great depth about the health benefits of a plant-based diet and the damaging effects of consuming animal products. (For a list of recommended books and further reading, see the Appendix, "Learn More about Plant-Based Living.") For the sake of brevity, I'll keep to the main points and most common myths here.

the dairy myth

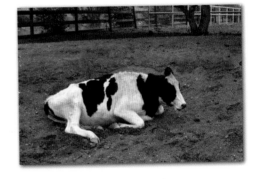

One of the biggest lies we've been told is that dairy is an essential source of calcium and the key to strong bones. Not only is milk *not* the best source of calcium, it wreaks havoc on our health and bones.

Here are just some of the facts that debunk the dairy myth:

» Greens and broccoli contain more calcium than milk.
» Dairy doesn't reduce fractures—it *increases* your risk of fracture by 50 percent![2]
» Worldwide, the incidence of osteoporosis correlates strongly with dairy consumption. Africa and Asia, for example, have both the lowest rates of osteoporosis and the lowest consumption of dairy, while places with the highest levels of dairy consumption (e.g., the United States) have the highest rates of osteoporosis. *Why?* Dairy actually leaches calcium from your bones![3]

» Dairy has been strongly linked to prostate cancer, acne, eczema, constipation, heart disease, strokes, obesity, sinus congestion, migraines, stomach issues, anemia, heartburn, type 1 and 2 diabetes, ear infections, irritable bowel syndrome, and many other conditions.

» More than 60 percent of the global population is lactose intolerant.[4] Scientists say we shouldn't even call lactose intolerance an allergy or a disease because that would imply the intolerance is abnormal.

» Dairy contains a naturally occurring hormone called insulin-like growth factor 1, which is one of the most powerful promoters of cancer growth ever discovered for breast, prostate, lung, and colon cancers.[5]

By consuming dairy, we're not only breast-feeding past infancy, we're also breast-feeding on a whole other species! No other species consumes the milk of *another* species. Dairy is super weird when you think about it!

---

the protein myth

All foods—including fruits and vegetables—contain protein, and many plant foods pack more protein than meat. For example, spinach and kale have nearly twice as much protein as beef, calorie for calorie.[6]

Does your meat eat other meat for protein? Nope! Most farm animals are herbivores. They develop their sought-after protein from plants. By eating plants, you're effectively removing the middleman.

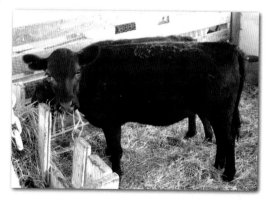

Point being, when you adopt a plant-based lifestyle, don't fret over protein. Absent special medical circumstances, you cannot be protein deficient unless you're calorie deficient, and then you're deficient in *everything* because you're starving.

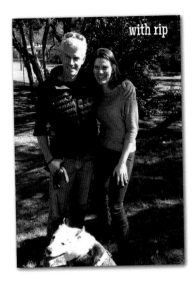
with rip

I especially love what my friend Rip Esselstyn, former professional triathlete and author of *The Engine 2 Diet*, says about protein deficiency: "Protein deficiency is so rare that I have never found a *single* person who knows the name of the medical condition that results from a serious lack of it in the diet." (If you're curious, the condition is called *kwashiorkor.*) According to the Academy of Sciences, Institute of Medicine, the recommended dietary allowance for both men and women is 0.8 grams of protein per kilogram of body weight (keep in mind this figure includes a fairly liberal margin for safety).[7] For a 150-pound person (about 68 kg) that would equate to nearly 55 grams per day. To put that amount in perspective, 1 tablespoon of peanut butter has 8.1 grams of protein. One cup of beans has 15 grams of protein, 1 cup of peas has 8 grams of protein, 1 cup of broccoli has 4 grams of protein, 1 cup rice has 5 grams of protein, and a baked potato has 3.4 grams of protein. In fact, you could literally eat nothing but potatoes all day and still exceed your daily protein needs!

THE "COMPLETE" PROTEIN MYTH

Plant proteins aren't "incomplete" or missing amino acids. Nor do you need to bind or pair various plant foods together to get "complete" proteins.[8] Your body pulls all the necessary building blocks (amino acids) it needs from *all* the foods you eat, even if you don't eat them at the same time or in the same meal.

The myths of incomplete protein and complementary protein can be traced back to the original (1971) publication of *Diet for a Small Planet* by Frances Moore Lappé. A sociologist—not a nutritionist or a medical doctor—Lappé later retracted her claims, stating that all plant foods do in fact contain all the essential amino acids, and that humans are virtually certain of getting enough protein from plant sources as long as they consume sufficient calories. Unfortunately, Lappé's initial misunderstanding about plant proteins persists.

Here's how it works: If you calculate the amount of essential amino acids provided by any single whole plant food or a combination of whole plant foods, you will find that when consumed as one's sole source of calories for a day, plant foods provide not only the daily minimum recommended requirement of essential amino acids, but provide far more.[9] In fact, it is virtually impossible to design a diet based on whole plant foods that is deficient in *any* of the amino acids, as long as the diet has enough total calories overall. (The only possible exception could be a diet based solely on fruit.)

THE ATHLETES' PROTEIN MYTH

Athletes and bodybuilders, plant-based or not, need more calories than the average person, but they do not need added concentrated sources of "nutrition."[i] Recent studies suggest we gain more muscle by consuming extra calories from carbohydrates or fats rather than from protein.[ii,10] Even protein powder manufacturers haven't been able to show a correlation between dietary protein and muscle mass, once daily minimums for nutrition are met.[11]

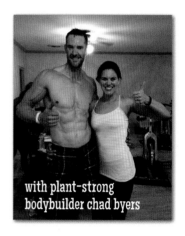

with plant-strong bodybuilder chad byers

the grass-fed myth

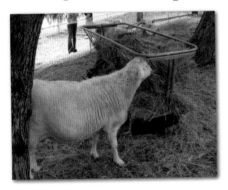

Animal products that are organic, "free-range," "humanely raised," and/or grass-fed remove some of the smaller problems with consuming animal products (such as the troubling effects of added hormones, steroids, chemicals, and antibiotics) but not the bigger issues. Cholesterol, animal protein, and fat (especially saturated fat) are the real problems with meat, dairy, and eggs, and those troublemakers exist no matter how the animal lived or died.[12]

---

i. Individuals who exercise for one hour or less generally do not need to increase their calories very much, if at all. If you find yourself losing weight (and you don't want to), bump up your calories. If you exercise for longer than one hour, adjust your calories to meet your caloric demands from exercise. There is no need to add any powder, shakes, and so forth, most of which are highly processed and unhealthy. Eat whole foods.

ii. The Academy of Nutrition and Dietetics estimates athletes need 10 to 12 percent of their total calories from protein, which is easily met on a whole food, plant-based diet. Agencies like this one also tend to recommend more than is actually necessary as a precaution.

DAVID: ONCE IMMOBILE & AN ADDICT, NOW A PLANT-BASED BODYBUILDER

june 2012

HH: Tell us a little bit about yourself and your history.

I am fifty-one and have been on a plant-based diet for almost a year. In the past, I have had significant physical trauma and was told I would always have pain, always be on meds, and never be able to exercise again. I did not walk for many months. It took almost a year to improve enough to walk a block, and I was up to 290 pounds.

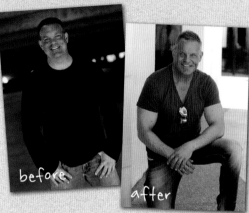

before

after

HH: Can you tell us a little bit about these traumas and surgeries?

I have had a series of physical traumas, several of which were very serious and life-threatening. At age eleven, while hiking, I climbed up on a boulder that (unbeknownst to me) was unstable. I fell and as I tried to get up, the 300-pound boulder fell on me, shattering my pelvis and pinning me in water. I had severe organ damage and did not walk for almost a year.

Thankfully I recovered, did karate, played lacrosse in high school and football in college, and lifted very heavy weights. I was benching more than 400 pounds, was a black belt in karate, and was pretty sure I was bulletproof. Then the lumbar discs started to go.

I have had nine spinal surgeries—ruptured lumbar discs were the first surgeries, followed by more than fifty epidurals, translaminals, facet injections, and other injections.

One night I got between a guy with a knife and his girl, who he was intent on killing. I suffered eight puncture wounds and a fourteen-inch laceration resulting in partial evisceration and a partial colectomy. I spent a month in the hospital.

Years later I had a fractured cervical vertebra and a full cervical fusion with a full titanium cage. Six surgeries in six months, along with a near fatal staph infection.

All these past traumas resulted in a variety of issues—addiction to pain pills and alcohol to name a couple.

Finally, in December of 2011, the scar tissue from the knife attack resulted in a rupture of my intestines. I was rushed into emergency surgery. After a twelve-inch incision from my solar plexus (upper abdomen) to my pubic bone, I was in the hospital for a month.

HH: Oh my goodness! Did you have any other medical issues or conditions outside of these physical ones and the addictions?

I ended up severely hypertensive (180/120 or so, resting pulse of 110) with lipidemia (lipids in the blood), arrhythmia (irregular heartbeats), chronic pain, and SIRS (systemic inflammatory response syndrome). I was on Norco, morphine, Soma, Flexeril, Ativan, Ambien, and metoprolol, among other meds.

I also had dangerously high triglycerides and VLDL (very-low-density lipoprotein) as well as cholesterol. I was on massive doses of pain and anti-inflammatory meds, sleeping pills, and muscle relaxers. Everything hurt.

HH: What brought you to a plant-based diet?

About a year ago I was diagnosed as celiac. I started reading a lot more about food. I started getting a Community-Supported

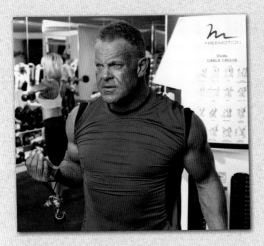

As a bodybuilder, I felt I needed a lot of animal protein, so I took *huge* amounts of whey—15 pounds a month. I spent $200 a month just on chicken breasts! I now use Sunwarrior Warrior Blend: pea, hemp, and rice proteins. I am stronger than ever—stronger than anyone at the UFC gym here (benching over 500 lb. and leg press over 1,400). I am leaner and faster, have increased my cardiac output, and am stronger than I have ever been in my life on a plant-based diet.

HH: Any closing comments or advice to bodybuilders and those thinking about switching their diet?

The switch to a plant-based diet has been a complete catharsis for me. I am a reborn soul. I am kinder, gentler, healthier, and happier. The most beautiful part of all of this has been a spiritual awakening. My anger and sarcasm are virtually gone.

UPDATE (summer 2014):

I am still plant-proud after four years. I am happy to report that I have not cheated once! I am still doing Muay Thai and lifting insanely heavy weights at the gym, and am very active in promoting the plant-based lifestyle.

I have recently signed with a new commercial and print talent agency, and hope to get some jobs! I was featured in Renaissance Club Sport's promotion campaign, and was on promotional materials, including a large poster that hung in the gym where I worked out. I was also selected to be a principal in UFC Gym's national print and video campaign, and was featured on several promotional pieces, including a large banner, featuring me, which also hangs in the gym where I work out. This is all very surreal to me, as I never would have guessed that I would be in good enough shape to be starring in any gym's campaign, but two of them? Sweet! I credit Lindsay's Happy Herbivore series with much of my success. I have also purchased several copies and mailed them to people I only know through Facebook, and for whom I thought the book would be useful. And it was, to each and every one of them. Go PLANTS!

Agriculture delivery. I heard Robert Lustig's lecture "Sugar: The Bitter Truth" and watched *Forks Over Knives*.

HH: Have you experienced any positive changes since adopting a plant-based diet?

As soon as I quit the arachidonic acid barrage (eggs, chicken, and whey protein), the changes started. The pain vanished. I am now off all meds. I have near perfect lab results and virtually no pain. I train twenty hours a week, spar in Muay Thai four days a week, lift, and do brutal high-intensity interval and CrossFit training as well.

HH: That's incredible! You went from a life of pain and immobility to being fit and active! Aside from these impressive changes and getting off the meds, have you experienced any other benefits?

I have lost 70 pounds and 7 inches off my waist, and went from a size 38 waist to a 31 in a year's time. I was 38 percent body fat—now I am 9 percent at 6'1" and 195 pounds. Blood pressure is 110/60, pulse 45. I am easily the strongest guy at my local UFC Gym and have maintained all of my lean muscle mass by eating only plants. The most flattering thing is when jaws drop when I say I am "vegan," as the common perception is not one of a man of my build.

HH: You're a bodybuilder. What is different about your diet now?

As Dr. T. Colin Campbell, Jacob Gould Schurman Professor Emeritus of Nutritional Sciences at Cornell University, has stated, "The adverse effects of animal protein . . . are related to their amino acid composition . . . This focus on amino acid composition of proteins is important because animal based protein will be the same regardless whether it is provided by grass-fed or feed lot fed animals."[13]

Switching to meat products labeled as organic, grass fed, "humanely raised," or "free range" does nothing to decrease the risk for diseases that remain the biggest killers in modern society.

the soy myth

Soy is perfectly safe, with three legitimate exceptions: (1) Some people are allergic to soy just as some people are allergic to corn or wheat, and those individuals should abstain from soy products; (2) individuals with certain medical conditions may need to avoid soy; and (3) genetically modified soy is not as healthy as organic soy, and highly processed soy foods such as imitation meat and soy cheese should be limited or avoided. However, this third point is true for *any* food. Organic, non-GMO, whole (unprocessed) foods are always preferable over their more processed or modified counterparts, soy or otherwise. (To demonstrate this point in lectures, I use the comparison of whole, organic corn to high-fructose corn syrup. See the difference?)

The pro-dairy, anti-soy scaremongers have done a great job at spreading numerous myths about the "dangers" of soy, but even their most reasonable-sounding arguments lack concrete evidence. If you look for solid proof to justify the soy myths, you won't find any. For example, the anti-soy scaremongers often accuse soy of raising estrogen in the body because soybeans contain isoflavones (also called phytoestrogens). Similar-sounding name, but isoflavones are not *estrogens*, and they have completely different effects on the body.

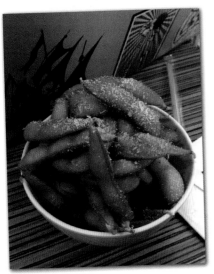

There is no research to support that soy enlarges breasts, causes infertility or cancer, or does whatever other wacky myth you may have heard. (It's interesting to note that sesame seeds, hummus, garlic, peanuts, flaxseeds, and other plant foods also contain isoflavones, and yet there's no hummus scaremongering.[iii] *Just sayin'*.) There is evidence, on the other hand, that dairy raises estrogen levels in the body.[14]

The way I see it, anti-soy scaremongers are a little like magicians: They're trying to focus your attention where it doesn't belong, so you can't see what's really happening. Luckily, magic isn't real—you can't make evidence disappear, or create evidence that doesn't exist out of thin air.

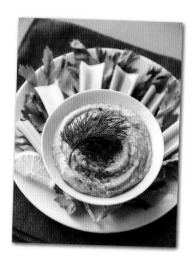

the oil myth

Olive oil and, more recently, coconut oil have had brilliant marketing campaigns. Their advertisements, masked as information, have most of us convinced that they are (1) heart healthy and (2) that we need these "good" fats (see "The 'Good Fat' Myth," next) to be healthy.

"The reality is that oils are extremely low in terms of nutritive value. They contain no fiber, no minerals, and are 100-percent fat calories. And above all, they contain saturated fat, which immediately injures the endothelial lining of the arteries when eaten," explains Dr. Caldwell B. Esselstyn Jr. of the world-renowned Cleveland Clinic and author of *Prevent and Reverse Heart Disease*.[15]

Consider this: A single tablespoon of oil has the same amount of fat as a candy bar, but the candy bar is arguably healthier since it provides other nutrients like fiber, protein, and carbohydrates, plus some vitamins and minerals where the oil does not—it's pure fat.

the "good fat" myth

All plant foods contain fat (even kale and bananas), so you get plenty of dietary "good" fat without adding high-fat foods like nuts or processed, highly concentrated

---

iii. For more information, read "Finally, the Truth About Soy," in Zen Habits, a blog by Leo Babauta (May 30, 2011). http://zenhabits.net/soy.

sources like oil. In the words of Dr. John McDougall, a physician and nutrition expert, "The fat you eat is the fat you wear… Fats (and oils) are the metabolic dollar stored for the day when food is no longer available. Even 'healthy oils' are moved from the spoon to the flesh with such efficiency that you should assume every drop you eat makes that journey."[16]

That said, active adults at a healthy weight without heart disease, type 2 diabetes, or other serious health conditions can generally enjoy high-fat whole plant foods such as nuts, seeds, and avocados sparingly. Children, on the other hand, need more fat for brain development, but those fats should still be whole fats like peanut butter or avocado. (See "Children and the Plant-Based Diet" for more information and resources.)

the fatty acids (or fish oil) myth

You don't need to eat fish or fish oil to get your omega-3s. (Fish, by the way, get *their* omega-3s from eating plants.)

Dr. Esselstyn explains, "It is difficult to be deficient in omega-3 if eating 1 to 2 tablespoons of flaxseed meal or chia seeds and green leafy vegetables at several meals. There is also research that suggests that those on plant-based nutrition become highly efficient in their own manufacture of omega-3."[17] Essentially, the body can convert the omega-3 fatty acid ALA (alpha-linolenic acid), found in plant foods, into the two omega-3 fatty acids found in fish: DHA (docosahexaenoic acid) and EPA (eicosapentaenoic acid).

Walnuts and flaxseed are excellent sources of omega-3s. Cloves, soybeans, tofu, kale, collard greens, hemp seeds, pumpkin seeds, chia seeds, and winter squash are other good sources of omega-3s.[18]

the mediterranean diet myth

The "Mediterranean diet"[19] is a multibillion-dollar-a-year branding business.[20]

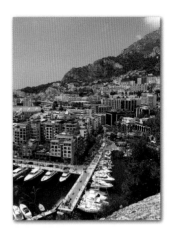

More than twenty (!) different countries border the Mediterranean Sea, and they all have completely different diets. Some eat fish, some don't. Some use olive oil, some don't...Which is it? It's whatever is convenient and can sell you something, that's what! By the way, the modern health statistics of most of these countries are as scary as ours.[iv] For example, in 2007, more than 45 percent of today's Italian population was overweight. The same was true for Portugal, Spain, and Greece, the last, as of this date, being the sixteenth fattest country in the world.[21] Whatever the "Mediterranean Diet" is, it doesn't appear to be working for them, either.

the vitamin and mineral deficiencies myth

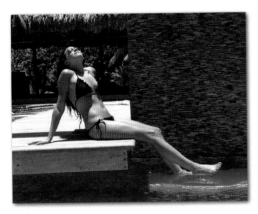

Deficiencies can (and do) happen on any diet, and sometimes those deficiencies are unrelated to diet. For example, we get vitamin D from the sun, so individuals in cold or overcast climates may need to supplement, regardless of diet.[22] Similarly, all women are susceptible to iron-deficiency anemia during their childbearing years because of blood loss from menstruation and increased blood demands during pregnancy.

---

iv. Most promoters of the myth point to studies from the 1940s and 1950s, a postwar time when most of the Mediterranean region was poor, and thus its people were eating a predominantly plant-based diet. As soon as these populations could afford rich foods, meats, and dairy, their obesity rates skyrocketed, along with incidences of heart disease and other diet-related illnesses.

When I was traveling through the Mediterranean to research *Happy Herbivore Abroad*, I found it fascinating that many traditional recipes now containing animal products were originally plant-based. On reflection it makes total sense: these cultural recipes were developed by peasants who were simply too poor to afford animal products. I also noticed that even in Italy olive oil was not used as generously or as abundantly as in America.

Being plant-based doesn't put you at greater risk for deficiency. All the essential vitamins and minerals we need exist in plant foods, in abundance, *and* plants are typically the richest source of these vitamins and minerals. Your garden is your pharmacy!

On the next page is a table that identifies plant-based sources of several key vitamins and minerals. The table is not comprehensive for all sources—I've only included the foods with the highest percentage daily value per serving of these vitamins and minerals.

Note that while the scale is from 0 to 100 percent, many plant foods exceed the daily value by four or more times (e.g., kale's vitamin K at 1327.6 percent). These supercharged numbers can make the other values seem smaller than they really are, however. For example, the vitamin E in sunflower seeds looks puny in comparison at 61.5%, even though sunflower seeds are the richest source there is for vitamin E, bar none.

Lastly, the richest source for any vitamin or mineral might also surprise you. For example, notice how oranges are not the richest source for vitamin C? Marketing magic, isn't it?

the vitamin B_{12} myth

Most doctors and nutritionists recommend supplementing a plant-based diet with vitamin B_{12} as a precaution, but B_{12} deficiency isn't strictly a vegan problem. Plenty of meat eaters test low for B_{12}, too, because vitamin B_{12} doesn't originate 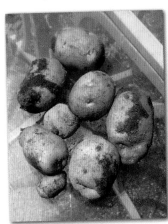 in plants *or* animals—it's found in dirt and made by microorganisms.[23]

Some meat may contain vitamin B_{12}, but only because the animal the meat came from ate plants (plants!) that were covered in dirt containing B_{12}.

You *could* do the same, and if you have access to organic produce from a farmer's market, eating a little dirt with your plants isn't a bad idea, but a B_{12} supplement is probably the more favorable option for most of us. Many foods, like cereals and soy milk, are fortified with B_{12} as well.[24]

PLANT-BASED SOURCES OF ESSENTIAL VITAMINS AND MINERALS

Percentages in the table are percent daily value. Serving sizes are typically 2 teaspoons of spices or herbs, 1 piece of fruit, 1 cup cooked greens, 1 cup raw vegetables.[25]

VITAMIN A	sweet potatoes (438.1%), carrots (407.6%), spinach (377.3%), kale (354.1%), collard greens (308.3%), turnip greens (219.6%), Swiss chard (214.3%), winter squash (214.3%), mustard greens (177%), romaine lettuce (163.7%)
VITAMIN C	papaya (313.1%), bell peppers (195.8%), strawberries (141.1%), broccoli (135.2%), pineapple (131.4%), brussels sprouts (126.6%), kiwifruit (120%), oranges (116.1%), cantaloupe (97.8%), kale (88.8%)
VITAMIN K	kale (1327.6%), spinach (1110.6%), collard greens (1045%), Swiss chard (715.9%), mustard greens (524.1%), brussels sprouts (194.7%), parsley (155.8%), romaine lettuce (120.4%), broccoli (115.5%)
VITAMIN B$_6$	potatoes (27%), sunflower seeds (23.5%), spinach (22%), bananas (21.5%), avocados (19%), bell peppers (13.5%), turnip greens (13%), summer squash (12.5%), shiitake mushrooms (12.5%), basil (7.7%), garlic (7.4%), cayenne pepper (7.1%), cauliflower (6.7%), mustard greens (6%)
VITAMIN E	sunflower seeds (61.5%), almonds (44.8%), spinach (18.7%), Swiss chard (16.5%), turnip greens (13.5%), papaya (11%), mustard greens (8.4%), collard greens (8.3%), asparagus (7.5%), bell peppers (7.2%), kale (5.6%), raspberries (5.4%), cayenne pepper (5.3%), tomatoes (4.9%)
IRON	soybeans (49.1%), lentils (36.6%), spinach (35.7%), tofu (33.7%), sesame seeds (29.1%), chickpeas (26.3%), lima beans (24.9%), olives (24.6%), navy beans (23.8%), Swiss chard (22%), thyme (19.2%), asparagus (15.9%), cumin (15.5%)
CALCIUM	tofu (39.6%), sesame seeds (35.1%), collard greens (26.6%), spinach (24.4%), turnip greens (19.7%), blackstrap molasses (11.8%), Swiss chard (10.1%), kale (9.36%), basil (5.9%), oregano (5.7%), thyme (5.3%), cinnamon (5.2%) (ANIMAL SOURCES HAVE COMPARABLE NUMBERS)

plant-based food pyramid

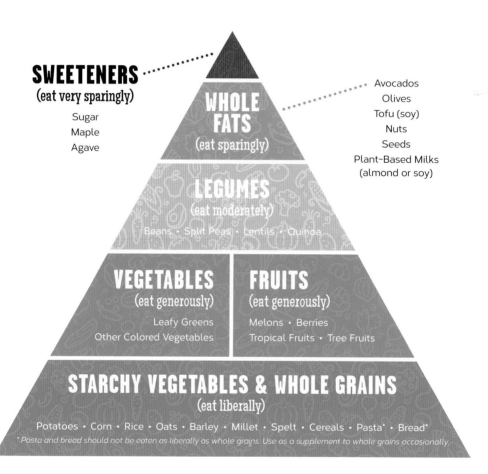

SWEETENERS
(eat very sparingly)

Sugar
Maple
Agave

WHOLE FATS
(eat sparingly)

Avocados
Olives
Tofu (soy)
Nuts
Seeds
Plant-Based Milks
(almond or soy)

LEGUMES
(eat moderately)

Beans • Split Peas • Lentils • Quinoa

VEGETABLES
(eat generously)

Leafy Greens
Other Colored Vegetables

FRUITS
(eat generously)

Melons • Berries
Tropical Fruits • Tree Fruits

STARCHY VEGETABLES & WHOLE GRAINS
(eat liberally)

Potatoes • Corn • Rice • Oats • Barley • Millet • Spelt • Cereals • Pasta* • Bread*

*Pasta and bread should not be eaten as liberally as whole grains. Use as a supplement to whole grains occasionally.

Use this revised food pyramid to guide
your plant-based diet.

CHRIS: FINALLY LOVING HIMSELF THANKS TO A PLANT-BASED DIET
october 2012

HH: You often describe your lifestyle before being plant-based as "self-abuse." Can you elaborate on that?

Being raised to "finish everything on my plate" before leaving the dinner table started what would become a disastrous habit. Growing up, I was constantly gorging on any food my heart desired. I ate every type of animal product, processed snack, soda pop, candy bar, et cetera. Whatever I was hungry for, I consumed—no holds barred.

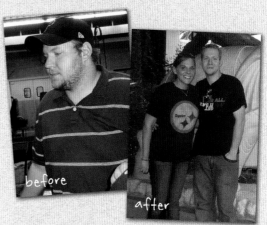

before

after

Examples of my meals include eating four or five Whopper Jrs. with onion rings and a milkshake for lunch, an entire pizza for dinner, and constant gas station snack-cake and cappuccino purchases. This was an everyday habit.

At the time, I wasn't aware of a problem with my behavior. Needless to say, I blew up. Eventually, I'd get sick of the weight and diet, but this was never a permanent solution. I jumped on multiple weight-loss bandwagons—Atkins, diet pills, exercise regimens, and so on. I'd lose pounds and then gain. I rode the weight-loss roller coaster for ten years.

HH: What happened? What made you change your diet?

I found myself at a tipping point when I was twenty-four. My skin was greasy and full of pus-filled boils. My joints hurt and it was hard to walk up stairs. I didn't even want to go out anymore. My doctor told me, "You're 320 pounds, your blood pressure is high, and you have high cholesterol. You can take pills for the rest of your life starting now or lose some weight." I knew that this was only the beginning of a road that probably would have killed me before I was forty. I "woke up" and decided that it was time to dramatically change course.

HH: What did you do?

I started by cutting down portions and that helped me get the weight-loss process rolling. If I cut something out of my diet,

I replaced it with something just a little bit healthier. Within one and a half years, I had lost about 80 pounds. I continued on this path, breaking the century mark of 100-pound weight loss and beginning an exercise program.

Then, I saw a movie that changed my life—*Food, Inc.* This started my journey into organic and whole foods, which continued as I learned from documentaries like *Forks Over Knives*, *The Future of Food*, *Food Matters*, and *Fat, Sick & Nearly Dead*. I also read *The RAVE Diet & Lifestyle*, *The China Study*, *Green Smoothie Revolution*, and more. The more plant-based foods I implemented in my lifestyle, the more my body transformed positively. I have more energy, glowing skin, and most of all—I LOVE MY TRUE SELF. I cut out animal products altogether at the age of twenty-six. I lost more than 130 pounds and reached a healthy weight of about 185.

HH: What is your life like now?

I'm healthier than I've ever been and I feel so ALIVE! I exercise regularly, have run half-marathons, and ran the Pittsburgh Marathon on May 4, 2014, finishing in 4:53:57!

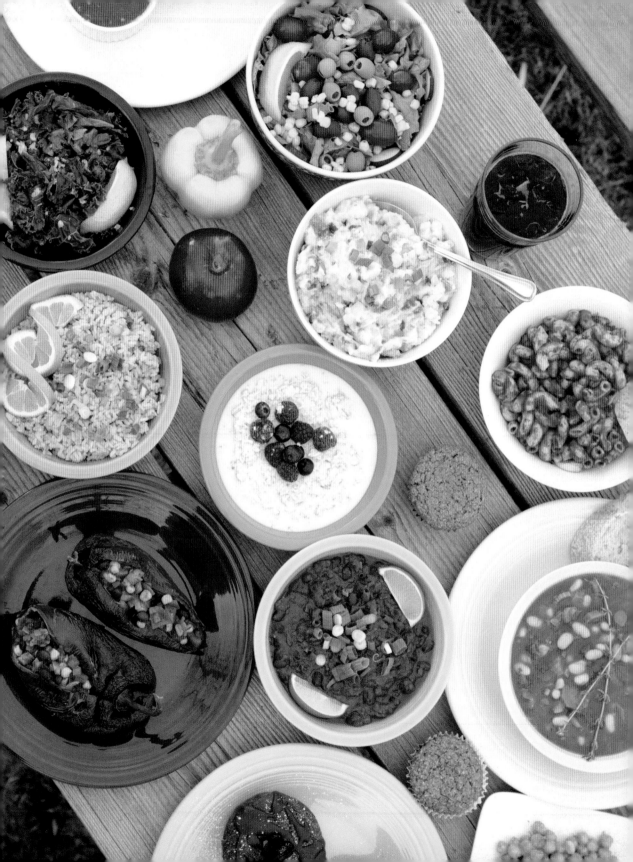

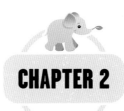

CHAPTER 2

why choose a plant-based diet?

*"Let food be thy medicine
and let medicine be thy food."*

—HIPPOCRATES—

When someone asks me why I am plant-based, I explain, "For my health, the plight of farm animals, the environment, the economy, and humanity," because putting plants on my plate greatly benefits all of those things. In fact, switching to a plant-based diet is the single most positive impact you can make on your health, the environment, and society. Following a plant-based diet is also a real, attainable solution to our national health crisis, and for many other crises around the world.

health benefits

chronic disease

Year after year, we hear that heart disease, type 2 diabetes, obesity, cancer, and other chronic illnesses are on the rise, but no one—not even the very health-care organizations dedicated to fighting or curing these illnesses—wants to point a finger at the Standard American Diet. Sure, one or two clear villains, like hydrogenated oils and saturated fats, are singled out, and we're told to cut back on this or that, eat more vegetables, and get more exercise; yet here we are, not only failing to improve, but sliding further downhill. In just twenty years, the United States went from not having *one* state with 20 percent obesity to not having one state that's *not* 20 percent obese, meaning the population of *every single state* is now at least 20 percent obese.

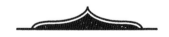

Health is more than the absence of disease. Health is a state of optimal well-being.

−WORLD HEALTH ORGANIZATION−

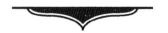

Even scarier, the current risk of being diagnosed with cancer for women is one in three. For men, it's one in two![1]

Most of us think our health is out of our control because we're victims of our genetics, and these organizations say little to make us feel otherwise. You hear almost nothing about prevention, except for costly medical prescreening exams that don't really *prevent* as much as identify problems earlier.

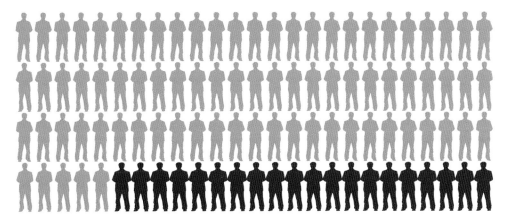

Today, in every U.S. state the population is 20 percent obese or more.

We also hear little about treatment that doesn't involve surgical intervention or medications, or treatments that actually *treat*—and *reverse*—the underlying problems, not just the symptoms.

Instead we're diagnosed with migraines, depression, or high cholesterol, and given a migraine pill, an antidepressant, or a statin with little thought as to why we ended up with migraines, depression, or high cholesterol in the first place or how we might *reverse* it. And most of what we hear about "cures" is only that the medical field is still racing to find one.

The truth is, we aren't hopeless victims to our genetics. We're victims of the Standard American Diet. As Dr. Esselsytn says in *Prevent and Reverse Heart Disease*, "Genes load the gun, but lifestyle pulls the trigger."[2]

The populations of the world with the healthiest and longest-living people follow diets that are primarily plant-based: rich in beans, whole grains, fruits, and vegetables, with zero processed foods, near-zero animal products, and low levels of oil and sugar.

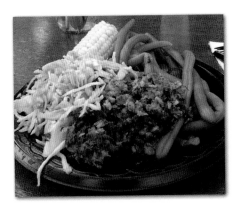

Numerous medical studies also show that heart disease, type 2 diabetes, most cancers, and a laundry list of other chronic illnesses like arthritis, fatigue, irritable bowel syndrome, acid reflux, chronic and seasonal allergies, eczema, psoriasis, autoimmune diseases, migraines, depression, and attention deficit

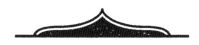

The food you eat can either be the safest and most powerful form of medicine or the slowest form of poison.

—ANN WIGMORE—

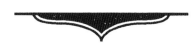

disorder can usually be prevented, treated, and *reversed* through diet.[3]

For example, Dr. Esselstyn has been reversing heart disease with a plant-based diet for more than twenty years. Dr. Dean Ornish of the Preventive Medicine Research Institute has also achieved similar results with his cardiac patients.

Similarly, Dr. Neal Barnard, a physician, clinical researcher, and founder of the Physicians Committee for Responsible Medicine in Washington, DC, and Dr. McDougall have both been reversing type 2 diabetes in their patients through a plant-based diet for decades, completely independent of each other.[4]

Additionally, in *The China Study*, the most comprehensive study in nutrition ever conducted, coauthor Dr. T. Colin Campbell shows how cancer growth can be turned on and off simply by adjusting the level of animal protein in one's diet. Campbell's findings have also been independently repeated by many of his peers, and numerous other independent studies continue to show a correlation between diet and modern disease.

Campbell says, "There are hundreds of detailed, comprehensive, well-done research studies that show a whole food, plant-based diet is best for preventing and reversing cancer, heart disease, type 2 diabetes, autoimmune diseases, strokes, Alzheimer's, osteoporosis, and many other diseases and illnesses."[5]

Dr. Neal Barnard adds, "When we break the meat seduction with a plant-based diet you reverse heart disease, lose weight, cancer risk drops by 40 percent, blood pressure drops, diabetes improves, and you will eliminate or reduce all medications."[6]

What about our technological advancements? None of the ultra-expensive high-tech advantages of the past fifty years have made a dent in overall rates of death and disease in developed countries. While today's medical advancements are much better at saving someone's life after an acute event like a car crash or a sudden heart attack than fifty years ago, we're not really better at preventing chronic degenerative diseases like heart disease and cancer, often called "disease of affluence," than we were in the 1950s.[7] Today, people are living *sicker* longer—but is that really living?

asthma and seasonal allergies

Itchy eyes, a scratchy throat, a stuffed nose, and the sneezes— seasonal allergies are the worst! But here's the good news: They can often be alleviated or totally eliminated with a plant-based diet!

When I first started helping others make the switch to a plant-based diet, I was focused on their weight loss, their blood pressure, whether they were able to reduce or get off their medications, and

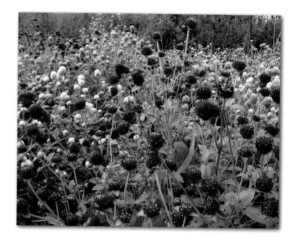

other serious medical issues and pains. I paid little attention to the "smaller" improvements such as my clients' sleeping better, having more clarity or less mental fog, or that they had stopped suffering from seasonal allergies.

In fact, it wasn't until my sister found relief from *her* allergies on a plant-based diet that I started looking over my clients' testimonials and seeing a new pattern. When I noticed a few had listed "no more seasonal allergies" as one of their many improvements, I started asking other clients if they'd noticed an improvement, too. (After all, since 50 million Americans suffer from seasonal allergies, including approximately 30 percent of adults and 40 percent of children, the odds were good that some of my clients were dealing with this, too.[8])

As more and more clients said, "You know, I hadn't realized it, but you're right, my seasonal allergies are gone," I wondered if there was science out there that could explain this. There is! It turns out that vegan and vegetarian diets have been studied since the mid-1980s and have been found to relieve both asthma and allergies!

To understand how a plant-based diet can help with seasonal allergies, we must first understand what seasonal allergies really are.

SEASONAL ALLERGIES

Seasonal allergies are caused by an inflammation of the mucous membranes lining your nasal passages. When you inhale airborne irritants from pollen, grass, flowers, and trees, your immune system detects them as invaders and sets off a

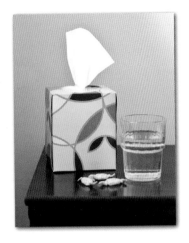

chain reaction of histamines and other chemicals, like leukotrienes, that result in inflammation, irritation, and discomfort. (Overproduction of leukotriene, particularly leukotriene D4, is a major cause of inflammation in asthma and allergic rhinitis.[i])

What does this chemical have to do with your diet? The production of leukotrienes is influenced by the presence of arachidonic acid in the body.[9] Arachidonic acid, or ARA, is a polyunsaturated omega-6 fatty acid that comes from animal foods like meat, dairy, and eggs.[ii] By eliminating these items from your diet, you can thereby reduce the presence of leukotrienes, a major cause of your inflammation and discomfort known as "seasonal allergies."

Several studies have also shown that people who eat more fruits and vegetables have reduced risk of asthma and seasonal allergies, presumably because of improved immune system functions from eating a healthy plant-centered diet.

For example, recent research shows that foods rich in vitamin E (like spinach, collard greens, kale, beans, carrots, celery, wheat germ, and nuts) can stop your immune system from overreacting to pollens or other allergens.[10] Quercetin, a flavonoid found in many fruits and vegetables, has also been shown to inhibit histamine and leukotriene release.[11]

But don't just take my word for it! I recently asked my fans to share their experiences with seasonal allergies, which you can read on my Facebook page (see https://www.facebook.com/HappyHerbivoreBlog/posts/10152431456748482).

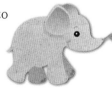

ORAL ALLERGY SYNDROME

About 30 percent of people who are allergic to pollen also have oral allergy syndrome, which means their immune system mistakenly sees a similarity between the proteins in some foods and the proteins in pollen.[12] In other words, for those who suffer from this syndrome, eating certain foods with pollen-like

---

i. Allergic rhinitis (more commonly called hay fever) is a common condition, with symptoms such as sneezing; stuffy nose; watery eyes; and itchiness of the nose, eyes, and mouth.

ii. ARA can also be found in vegetable oils (another reason to avoid them), but ARA in the human body usually comes from dietary animal sources.

characteristics can make their bodies react as if they were inhaling pollen.

Foods with these similar "trigger" proteins include apples, cherries, pears, apricots, kiwis, plums, and nuts. If you have an allergy to pollen, avoiding these foods may help. (Note: Cooking or peeling these foods can help avoid a reaction for some people.)

Individuals with a ragweed or other weed pollen allergy are also advised to avoid melons, bananas, cucumbers, and sunflower seeds, since these foods are from the same plant family and may cause a reaction when consumed.

NATURAL RELIEF

In addition to eliminating animal foods and eating a purely plant-based diet (and avoiding some plant foods if you have oral allergy syndrome), there are other natural ways to relieve seasonal allergies. For example, using a neti pot and drinking stinging nettle tea are other holistic, plant-based remedies.

ASTHMA

About one in twelve Americans has asthma, a chronic lung disease that narrows and inflames the airways. People with asthma may experience wheezing, chest tightness, shortness of breath, or coughing, particularly at night or early in the morning.[13]

While there is no cure for asthma, and the exact cause is still unknown,[14] we do know that a higher body weight or BMI increases the risk of asthma in both adults and children.[iii] For example, obese women have a 50 percent higher rate of asthma compared to non-obese women.[15]

Childhood diet has also been linked to asthma prevalence, but adult diet has been linked to asthma *severity*.[16] For example, recent reviews and studies have implicated arachidonic acid (found in animal products and vegetable oils) as a possible risk factor for asthma. (Plus, as mentioned, ARA increases production of leukotrienes, and overproduction of leukotrienes is a major cause of inflammation in asthma.)[17]

In addition, food-induced bronchospasm—constriction of the muscles in the walls of the bronchioles, the passageways that convey air from the main

---

iii. Obesity is an independent factor of asthma. Obesity mechanically compromises proper lung and airway function, which is associated with asthma-related inflammation.

bronchi deep into the lungs—occurs with the intake of certain allergenic foods (milk, eggs, peanuts, wheat, soy, legumes, and turkey) in 2 to 24 percent of people with asthma.[18]

Interestingly, asthmatic adults also show an increase in airway restriction after eating a meal high in animal fat and calories, but low in nutrients.[19] On the upside, several studies have found positive relationships between higher fruit and vegetable intake and reduced risk for asthma.[20] For example, the Nurses' Health Study found women in the highest quintile of vitamin E intake from food (not supplements) had a 47 percent lower risk of adult-onset asthma.[21] Similarly, vitamins C and E have been shown to significantly improve exercise-induced asthma.[22]

Moreover, in a study of nearly 28,000 people, vegetarian (and particularly vegan) women reported fewer incidences of asthma than non-vegetarian women.[23] One theoretical explanation is the absence of potential triggers of asthma (particularly meat, dairy, and eggs) and the ARA in the vegetarian and vegan women's diets. Similarly, a smaller clinical trial of asthma patients following a vegan diet also noted significant improvements in lung capacity and reduced needs for medications after one year on a vegan diet.[24]

Deana Ferreri, PhD, of the Nutritional Education Institute says, "A high-nutrient diet floods the body with protective micronutrients, reduces inflammation, and promotes weight loss—allowing the body to resolve the risk factors for asthma." She continues, "Dr. Joel Fuhrman has had much success using a [predominately plant-based] high-nutrient diet to treat patients with asthma—many recover completely and no longer need asthma medication."[25]

While additional research and clinical trials are needed to fully investigate the role of diet in asthma, the research we do have encourages more plant foods (and no animal foods and no oils) as both a preventive measure and a possible treatment for asthma.

hidden food allergies and sensitivities

When most of us think of food allergies, we think of a person who, after eating, has stomach distress, or in extreme cases, goes into anaphylactic shock, which is both serious and life threatening. But food allergies, intolerances, and sensitivities can be more hidden, causing a wide range of symptoms such as fatigue, skin issues (such as rashes, hair loss, hives, or eczema), nasal congestion, mood swings,

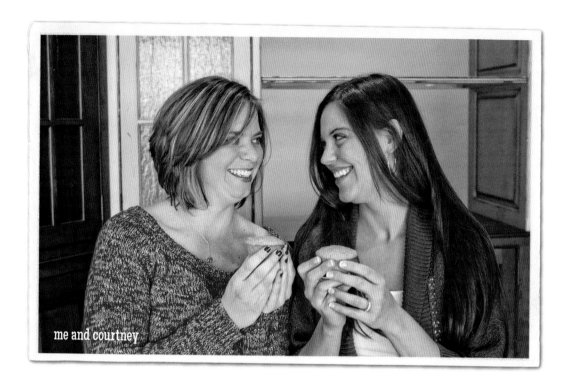
me and courtney

depression, headaches, gastrointestinal issues (such as diarrhea or constipation), canker sores, and other unpleasantries.

My sister Courtney's allergy story is one of my favorites to tell. For years she was stuffed up and unable to breathe fully. Eventually, her restricted airway started interfering with her sleep. Courtney would constantly wake up throughout the night, and in the morning her mouth would be dry and painful. When her nose finally became completely blocked, she called her doctor to schedule an appointment. The receptionist on the other end asked how long Courtney had been sick—that's how stuffed up she sounded! Courtney explained she wasn't "sick," she just couldn't breathe.

At the doctor's office, Courtney's nasal cavities were so swollen and blocked that the specialist wasn't even able to use a nasal endoscope, a small, thin viewing tube, to find the problem.

Prior to this appointment, though, Courtney had been seeing her regular physician, who suspected her stuffed nose was the result of an allergy. After several rounds of allergy testing, Courtney was diagnosed as allergic to grass, black pepper, and cottonseed. She was prescribed two allergy medications (one "indoor" for the foods, one "outdoor" for the grass), told to avoid her allergy "triggers," and sent home.

Unfortunately, even with strict abstinence from black pepper and cottonseed oil (which you can find in some tortilla chips and peanut butters) and diligent use of her medications, Courtney's condition only worsened, which is why she sought the help of a specialist.

The specialist gave Courtney a handout on cottonseed allergies, which suggested she avoid conventional (nonorganic) produce, since fruits like apples are sometimes polished with cottonseed oil, and milk, since cows are fed cotton-seed cakes. (Interestingly, it didn't tell her to avoid beef!) Courtney reluctantly complied and continued with her medications, but she still didn't feel better, until she came to visit me.

While I generally try not to push my lifestyle on my family, I do keep a vegan home, so I told my sister that she was free to eat however she wanted at restaurants, but that all the meals I'd be making at home would be plant-based.

To my sister's credit, she tried everything I made for her and genuinely seemed to enjoy the vegan-friendly restaurants I took her to. The entire week she was there, I only remember seeing her eat chicken once!

Then, the most amazing thing happened: Courtney's nose started to clear and she could breathe a little bit better. Of course it must be the very clean air of New York City, right?

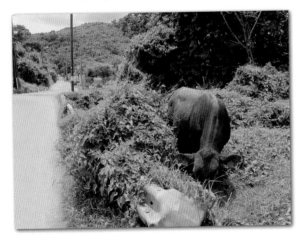

As soon as Courtney went home to Florida, her nose started acting up again, and she wondered if it was all the grass. She knew she was allergic, and the specific kind of grass she was allergic to is all over Florida, but if the meds weren't helping, was she going to have to move to Arizona?!

That's when her mind drifted back to the cottonseed pamphlet. It told her to avoid dairy because the cottonseed the cow eats will come out in its milk. Well, she thought, why wouldn't cottonseed also be stored in its muscles (beef)? After a little more digging,

Courtney discovered cottonseed *would* be stored in their muscles, and that it's fed to nearly all livestock—not just cows!

At that moment, Courtney decided to go completely plant-based to resolve her allergies. She told me, "I thought I was able to avoid cottonseed by looking at ingredients of something, but where do you get the ingredients of a filet? I never thought that what the cow was eating I also was eating. It gave a realistic meaning to 'you are what you eat.'"

Within two weeks, all of Courtney's allergy symptoms were gone! She was breathing completely normally and stopped taking her food-allergy medication.

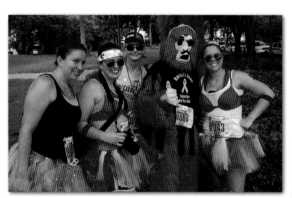 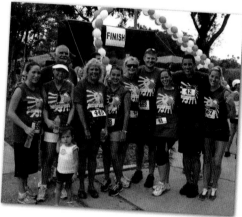

courtney's a regular 5k-er now!

A little while later Courtney completed her first 5K, and I sobbed with delight. To see her complete the 5K for charity that she had always wanted to run but couldn't before, because it was too difficult with her labored breathing, was one of the happiest and proudest days of my life. (And if you're wondering about that grass allergy, she eventually went off that medication as well. It wasn't the plant-based diet that necessarily helped, but a daily local honey regimen has done wonders for her.)

It's over four years since, and Courtney is still plant-based, still off all of her allergy medications, and still breathing at full capacity. (And I'm still one very proud sister, too!)

The reasons why some people are allergic to some things (cottonseed in Courtney's case and broccoli in mine) and others are not is still a big puzzle in the science community, but we're creeping closer to an answer. Dr. McDougall notes,

"Most scientists think that susceptibility to allergens may be due to an inherited predisposition. However, considerable evidence indicates that introducing certain foods (including cow's milk) too soon into an infant's diet, at the time when its intestinal tract and immune systems are still immature, may provoke responses in its tissues that will lead to symptoms of allergy later in life. Similarly, respiratory allergies and skin problems may be started at that tender age, when the infant's immune responses are unable to cope properly with the alien allergens."[26]

If you have a chronic issue or annoyance that persists even after you've adopted a totally plant-based diet, the ultimate and best test for identifying your trigger is an elimination diet. For more information about starting an elimination diet, see "Sensitivities and Food Allergies" in chapter three (page 70).

> If you're ready to start an elimination diet, check out my fourteen-day elimination diet plan (it's egg-free, dairy-free, meat-free, fish-free, soy-free, wheat-free, gluten-free, corn-free, nut-free, yeast-free, sugar-free, oil-free, and completely unprocessed!) at www.happyherbivore.com/elimination-diet.

Admittedly, I ate broccoli for years thinking it was "good for me," and broccoli is absolutely a healthy, nutritious food, but I feel a whole lot better now with broccoli *out* of my diet. An elimination diet also helped me discover that while I can eat bananas and oranges just fine, I cannot eat oranges and bananas *together*. Everyone's gut has its own little quirks!

obesity and weight loss

Obesity has become a global epidemic—the World Health Organization formally recognized obesity as a global epidemic in 1997.[27] It's also a hard, and often sensitive, topic to talk about. For example, at conferences I can't say "Obesity is an epidemic in this country" without someone accusing me of "fat shaming" or being a "sizeist," so let's get that out of the way first. Healthy and unhealthy people come in all shapes and sizes, and how someone may look on the outside is no indicator of their true health. I also personally believe that everyone should feel beautiful and proud of their amazing bodies, and should never *ever* feel like they have to change themselves or their body to fit some other person's arbitrary definition of beauty. Also, we should never do something to ourselves just to make someone else happy or more comfortable. This is your life and your body!

That said, "obesity"[iv] is a medical condition (classified by the American Medical Association as a disease in 2013[28]) that carries adverse effects such as reduced life expectancy and/or increased risk for serious diet-related diseases such as cardiovascular disease, hypertension, stroke, type 2 diabetes, and certain forms of cancer.[29] Obesity is also a leading preventable cause of death worldwide, with increasing rates in adults and children. My point is, it doesn't matter how beautiful, how confident, or even how healthy someone is—carrying around significant excess body fat is taxing on their organs and joints. If we want to be as healthy as possible in terms of reducing risks for *other* diseases, and maximizing our potential life expectancy (while enjoying the highest quality of life possible, too!), the excess weight has to come *off*.

Presently, the United States has the second-highest obesity rate in the developed world (after Mexico). While obesity was relatively scarce for centuries, by 1962, 45 percent of adult Americans were overweight, and 13 percent were obese. Today, 69 percent of adult Americans are overweight (including those who are obese), and 35.1 percent of the adult population is obese.[30]

Even more worrisome is the growing prevalence of overweight and obese children. The obesity rate among children ages 2–19 has steadily increased over the last decade. Today, 18.4 percent of children ages 12–19, 18 percent of children ages 6–11, and 12.1 percent of children ages 2–5 are obese.[31]

It's time to have a real conversation about obesity (and weight loss) as a society and without supercharged emotions, stigmas, or defensiveness.

why are we obese?

According to the *American Journal of Medicine*, the worldwide prevalence of overweight people is directly related to the percentage of fat in their diet.[32] This means the cause of obesity is not due to physical inactivity, personal weakness, a slow

---

iv. In the United States, obesity is defined as a body mass index (BMI) of 30 or greater, though many medical professionals feel BMI is not always the most helpful tool in determining obesity, since some people with a BMI above 30 can be perfectly healthy (and often very muscular), while others with a BMI below 30 can have dangerous levels of body fat.

metabolism, or a genetic curse. (While genetic factors *can* contribute to obesity, only a limited number of cases are due primarily to genetics.[33])

Evidence to support the view that some obese people gain weight due to a slow metabolism is also rather limited. On average, obese people have a greater energy expenditure than people who are not obese, due to the sheer amount of energy required to maintain an increased body mass.[34] Their metabolism is not slower, and they often burn more calories. Weight gain in the United States over the past thirty years is almost exclusively due to changing our eating habits, not a lack of physical activity.[35]

"The obesity epidemic is not caused by inactivity, bread, rice, gluttony, weak will, or a bad childhood. It is caused by a tsunami of unhealthful foods, and one of the worst, perhaps surprisingly, is cheese," explains Dr. Neal Barnard.[36]

The modern Western diet is also filled with "magic foods," highly palatable, energy-dense foods that are rich in fat and sugar—a dynamic duo that makes modern foods irresistible, incredibly addictive, and super illusionists! These magic foods, as the authors of *The Pleasure Trap* call them, interfere with our natural ability to read hunger signals and sense satiety, thereby leading us to overconsume. (Learn more about magic foods and food addiction in chapter six; see page 153.)

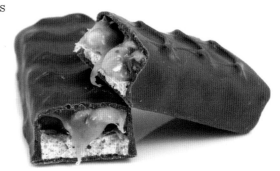

WHAT ABOUT CHEESE?

Going back to Dr. Barnard's earlier explanation, regarding cheese being one of the worst foods when it comes to obesity, he elaborates, "In 1909, the average American consumed only 3.8 pounds of cheese in a year's time. Today, that number is pushing 34 pounds. That's an increase of 30 pounds per person this year, next year, and again the year after that, thanks to the combined promotional efforts of government and industry. Of those extra 30 pounds of cheese we are stuffing into our mouths every year, it would only take one or two to stick in order to explain the entire weight problem in America. Of course, there are other co-conspirators in the obesity epidemic, too, notably the rise in meat and sugar consumption."[37]

FINDING A CURE

Obesity can be prevented and successfully treated in most individuals through a low-fat, low-sugar, no-oil, plant-based diet.

Reducing dietary fat (primarily found in meat, fish, dairy, eggs, and oils) is key. Not only does fat have twice as many calories per gram as protein and carbo-hydrates (9 calories per gram of fat vs. 4 calories per gram of protein or carbo-hydrate), it offers very little satisfaction for the hunger drive.[38] Dietary fat also promotes passive overconsumption of energy (food), which results in fat *storage* rather than fat oxidation.[39] (A reduced propensity to oxidize fat is a major risk for weight gain.[40])

This is why the prevalence of excess weight worldwide is directly linked to the percentage of fat in the diet,[41] and why low-fat diets continue to promote moderate weight loss in study after study. As you learned in "The 'Good Fat' Myth" section (p. 31), the fat you eat is the fat you wear—it literally goes from your lips to your hips! By eating a low-fat diet, you reduce your rate of fat ingestion and increase satiety through caloric density.

ENERGY DENSITY

Caloric density or energy density refers to the concentration of calories in a portion of food. For example, 2 tablespoons of nuts have the same amount of calories as two *cups* of cantaloupe. Nuts are high in energy density (lots of calories squeezed in a small package) while cantaloupe, like many other fruits and vegetables, is loaded with water 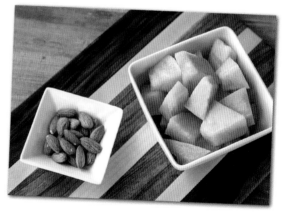 and fiber, which makes it much lower in energy density.

Flour, sugar, and oil (aka the three main ingredients in most processed foods) are all extremely energy dense.

Individuals who consume foods that are lower in energy density and higher in water and fiber, such as salads, soups, vegetables, and fruits, instead of foods high in energy density, experience early satiety, which spontaneously decreases food intake. This strategy has produced weight loss in several clinical studies.[42]

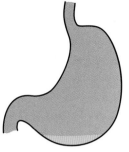

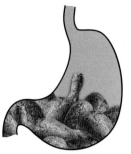

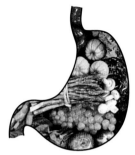

**400 calories
of oil**

**400 calories
of chicken**

**400 calories
of vegetables**

caloric density comparison

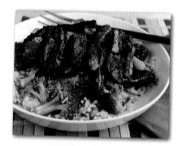

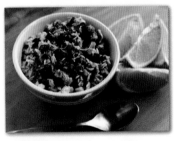

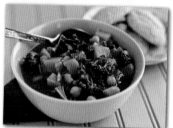

a few dishes from my
7-day meal plans!

I also see it every day with my 7-Day Meal Plan users (www.getmealplans.com). Energy density is the principle on which I base the meal plans. I get more e-mails about how *stuffed* everyone is from our big portions than I do from people who are still hungry. In fact, no one ever complains that they are still hungry! Our users cannot believe how much food they can eat for 1,200-plus calories.

The 7-Day Meal Plans (http://www.getmealplans. com) are so filling because they center around this energy density concept: **more food, fewer calories**. If you focus on selecting foods with a low-energy density, you can worry less about how much of them you're eating *and* you'll lose weight without ever feeling hungry or deprived.

More importantly, because you can eat larger portions of food and feel satiated this way, you'll stick with it. After all, that's one of the reasons why "diets" don't work long-term. The food portions are too small and you feel limited or hungry, or both. Eating a low-fat, plant-based diet is all about abundance, *not* deprivation. (Just another reason why I call getting on the plant-based highway to health a lifestyle choice and not a diet!)

In fact, results of the New Dietary Interventions to Enhance the Treatments for Weight Loss (NewDIETs) Study in late 2013 revealed that plant-based diets show more weight loss without caloric restriction. When results of this study were presented to The Obesity Society, lead researcher Brie Turner-McGrievy, PhD, of the University of South Carolina, remarked, "Many researchers agree that vegan eating styles are tied to lower BMI, lower prevalence of type 2 diabetes, and less weight gain with age."[43]

Dr. Turner-McGrievy continued, "This is the first randomized study that directly compares how vegan, vegetarian, and omnivorous dietary patterns that do not emphasize caloric restriction can impact body weight. We found that participants consuming vegan and vegetarian diets lost an average of 8.2 to 9.9 pounds over eight weeks while those consuming some meat lost 5.1 pounds."[v,44]

Randomized trials in 2005 also showed that low-fat vegan diets promoted greater weight loss than typical low-fat diets, while improving plasma lipids, insulin sensitivity, and other measured improvements.[45]

Learning about energy density and the plant-based diet changed my life and approach to food forever. If you have a voracious appetite like me, or you enjoy eating a lot of food (also like me), or you need to feel overly satiated in order to be able to avoid unhealthy, energy-dense treats (still like me!), then eating foods lower in energy density but higher in water and fiber will make a huge difference in your waistline. (Fiber intake is also inversely associated with body weight and body fat.[46])

Many studies have also widely reported that vegetarians and vegans tend to be slimmer than omnivores. For instance, Dr. Micheal Gregor, on his website nutritionfacts.org, has a great video in which he gives an overview of the first study done on thousands of vegans (it compared their BMIs to those of vegetarians, flexitarians, and omnivores.)[47]

the global impact of a plant-based diet

The relationship between animal agriculture and global resource depletion is well documented. For starters, in a 2010 report, the United Nations urged a

---

v. Mean (SD) percent weight loss (in pounds) was significantly different among the five groups (vegan, −4.8 ± 2.1%; vegetarian, −4.8 ± 3.2%; pesco-vegetarian, −4.3 ± 1.8%; semi-vegetarian, −3.7 ± 2.3%; omni-vegetarian, −2.2 ± 2.0%; intention-to-treat analysis, p > 0.05).

global shift toward a meat- and dairy-free diet. In the report, the United Nations concluded that meat and dairy production is severely damaging to the environment and requires significantly more resources than plant-based food production, the clear implications being that a vegan diet is vital to save the world from hunger, from fuel poverty, and from the worst impacts of climate change.[48] This report came after a 2000 World Health Organization report stating that one in every three people was suffering from malnutrition as a result of rapid population growth, diminished land, water, and energy resources.[49]

world hunger

Did you know:

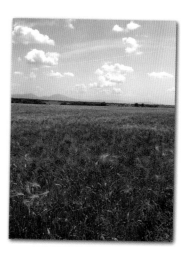

» Six million children in the world will die from starvation this year, and 1.1 billion people in the world are considered malnourished or suffer from hunger.[50]

» The United States could feed 800 million people with the amount of grain fed to livestock raised for meat. If those grains were exported, it would boost the U.S. trade balance by an estimated $80 billion![51]

» One acre of land can produce 165 pounds of meat or *twenty thousand pounds* of potatoes.[52]

Switching to a plant-based diet is by far the most impactful choice you can make toward ending world hunger.

water resources

Did you know:

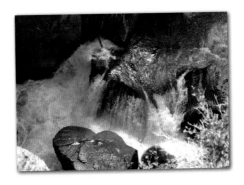

» Animal agriculture is a leading consumer of water resources in the United States. Studies vary, but beef production requires from 2,464 to 12,000 gallons of water for every *1 kilogram* of food. Broiler chickens require up to 3,500

liters per kilogram. In comparison, soybean production uses as little as 2,000 liters of water per kilogram; rice, 1,912 liters; wheat, 900 liters; and potatoes, only 500 liters.[53, 54]

» The amount of water needed to produce *1 pound* of beef is the same amount of water you would use, in total, if you took a shower every day for six months.[55]

» In 2005, only 13 percent of fresh water was used for domestic purposes, including showers, flushing toilets, washing cars, and watering lawns, according to the United States Geological Survey.[56]

» Water shortages due to droughts are already a serious problem in the western and southern U.S. states. Wells are going dry, water tables are dropping, and our aquifers are diminishing.[57]

Switching to a plant-based diet is by far the most impactful choice you can make to conserve water.

> **Change starts when someone sees the next step.**
>
> —WILLIAM DRAYTON—

fossil fuels

Did you know:

» Animal protein production requires more than *eight* times as much fossil-fuel energy than production of plant protein.[58]

» Averaged together, animal protein production requires 28 kilocalories of fossil fuel for every *1 kilocalorie* of protein produced, compared to plant proteins like tofu, for example, which requires 2.2 kilocalories. (Beef and lamb require the most energy at 54:1 and 50:1, respectively.[59])

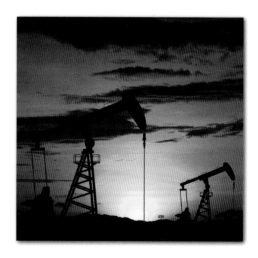

Switching to a plant-based diet is by far the most impactful choice you can make to conserve fossil fuels.

 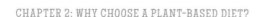

RUSS: LOST 100 POUNDS ON A PLANT-BASED DIET

october 2013

HH: What spurred your change? What made you get healthy?

About two years ago, I looked in the mirror and did not like what I saw. I went from my normal size 34 jeans to size 38, and they were getting too small. I knew I had to do something. I was also on four different medications, including one for high blood pressure, one for high cholesterol, one for high triglycerides, and finally, one for depression. I knew I had to make a change. But I also knew I had a few months of major holidays ahead of me. So I decided to wait until February 20, 2012, to start my diet.

Seeing how I still had six months before I was going to *start*, I'm not sure everyone believed I would really diet. After all, I was putting it off for so many months. However, my brother, wife, and mother knew I could.

HH: How'd you learn about the plant-based diet and lifestyle?

In the months before my start date, I watched the movie *Forks Over Knives*—I got excited! Then I learned about *The Engine 2 Diet*, and as a former volunteer firefighter, it hit home. Next I got my first book, *The Kind Diet*. I got even more excited, but could I really eat this way? I'm a great cook, and like everyone around me, I loved to eat meat. Also, I would drink half a gallon of 1 percent milk each day. Could I really do this? I was still not sure. Maybe I could just cut back and eat less.

Next I found The Happy Herbivore via the internet. I checked out Lindsay's website

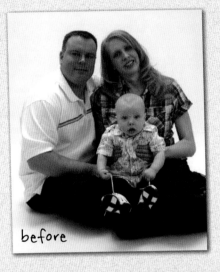

before

and got really excited. I ordered my first of her books, *The Happy Herbivore Cookbook*—I loved it. Keep in mind, it is still not yet February 20, but it was getting close. I started doing a little shopping, making small changes in my day-to-day diet, and then came the Big Day! February 20, 2012, had arrived.

HH: How'd you feel? Did you switch to a 100 percent plant-based diet that day?

I was scared! I'd hyped this diet up so much, could I really live up to it? On the first day, I did a lot of things with my Vitamix!!! I love that blender. I am going to confess, the first ten days were hard for me but by day eleven, this was not only easy, it was fun! Then I started doing a little more from the cookbooks.

HH: Did you experience any benefits?

I was down 20 pounds in the first two or three months! That got me really, really excited and I went hardcore. "I can do this, I really think I can," I told myself. I then got my next book, *Everyday Happy Herbivore*. Then I was really cooking!

I forgot to mention that at the start of my diet I was around 279 pounds! After a few months I was down 40 pounds to about 239 pounds! I had not seen that weight in over fourteen years.

HH: I've heard that you have inspired other family members to adopt a plant-based diet. Tell us about that.

Around the time I'd lost 40 pounds, I took a trip to see one of my brothers and his partner in Pennsylvania. The only problem was I had to go shopping so I could have things to make and eat.

They could not believe how good I looked and how much I had lost. His partner, who had been going to the gym for almost two years and lost 10 pounds, was excited. I showed them some of the simple things I ate. When I left, I had overshopped, so I left some things behind. My brother's partner then started to try some of my food and went on a vegan diet. Now they both look great. I can tell that my brother's partner has lost weight. She was just here visiting us a few weeks ago and looks great!

HH: Tell us more about what happened after you became plant-based.

I never went to the gym to lose this weight, but I sure watched what I ate and I was faithful to my new . . . diet? No, this was no longer a diet, it was a lifestyle change. Now I'm off all my cholesterol and blood pressure medication, because my numbers are perfect!

I lost 97 pounds in a little over a year. I'm now 182 pounds! I look and feel great. I'm now wearing size 30 jeans, and they are not tight. I think I could fit into size 29s. And I just got my copy of *Happy Herbivore Abroad*!

HH: Anything else you'd like to add?

I just want to give special thanks to Lindsay S. Nixon, Rip Esselstyn, Alicia Silverstone, the folks at *Forks Over Knives*, and so many others! Thanks for giving me the foundation for my new healthy life! Without all of you, I would not be where

I am today. My sincerest thanks to you all. I hope my story helps and motivates others.

UPDATE (summer 2014)

I'm now a year older and still doing great!!! I lost a total of around 130 pounds but now sustain a loss of just around 115 pounds. I really was too thin at one point. Who knew that I would ever say that?

Although I still am a vegan, I eat a few things with a little oil in them. I have to tell you, this is really life changing. I have no doubt that had I stayed on the path I once walked that I would not be around to see my young kids grow up. I have two boys: Hayden, who is five; and Preston, who is three. I also have my lovely wife, Debbie, who is thirty-seven. I want to be sure that I'm here for them, as I think they need me as much as I know I need them. I'm now forty-four and feel better than I have in ten years.

I no longer use the CPAP machine, and

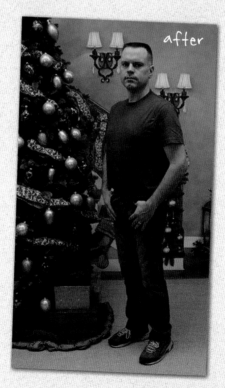

after

am still off most of my meds, but I did return to one for anxiety. I just did not function well without it. It has nothing to do with diet, just my stressful life.

I would like to thank everyone for the great support and to also tell Lindsay thanks for the tools and support, and I hope one day to meet her in person to give her a really big hug!

So, for those of you who don't think you can, or who think it has to be hard, I just want to tell you that yes, you can, and it's really easy. You start to look at food a little differently than you had in the past, but in a good way.

other environmental factors

Did you know:

» "Livestock production accounts for 18 percent of global greenhouse gas emissions—which is more than all of the world's automobiles combined," according to the Food and Agriculture Organization.[60]

» About 90 percent of U.S. cropland is losing topsoil at a rate thirteen times *higher* than what is considered sustainable. While both plant and animal agricultural practices are to blame, the loss of soil from plant farming is roughly six times slower than the loss from meat farming, *and* most of the crops grown are food for livestock![61]

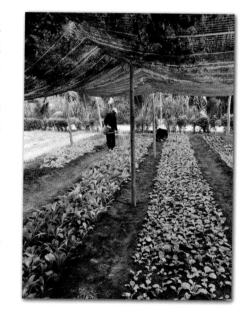

» Livestock farms pollute our clean water stores and oceans, creating "dead zones" with no aquatic life. Additionally, fecal runoff contains dangerous pathogens like *Salmonella* and *E. coli,* which often end up on crops. According to the Natural Defense Council, "more than forty diseases can be transferred to humans through manure."[62]

» The U.S. Environmental Protection Agency estimates that animal agriculture accounts for 50 to 85 percent of total human-made ammonia volatilization in the United States. Among the many potential impacts of ammonia are damage to our surface waters and crops, and human respiratory problems. Ammonia also causes acid rain.[63]

» The meat industry is the number-one source of methane[vi] throughout the world, releasing over 100 million tons per year.[64]

» According to the Nature Conservancy, every second of every day one football field's worth of rain forest is destroyed to make room for more cattle ranching.[65] The meat from those animals is then exported to the United

---

vi. Methane gas traps heat in the atmosphere, causing the earth's temperature to rise. Many experts believe the increase in methane is a leading cause of global warming.

States for fast-food hamburgers. (According to the Rainforest Action Network, 55 square feet of tropical rain forest—the size of a small kitchen—is permanently destroyed to make a single hamburger.[66])

» Rain forest destruction also causes untold losses of biodiversity. Up to thirty different plant species, one hundred different insect species, and

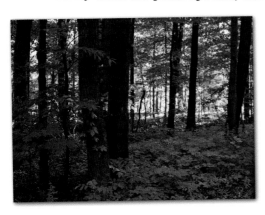

dozens of bird, mammal, and reptile species live within a single square foot of rain forest. All of these species are destroyed during deforestation, along with the trees that provide oxygen and filter air pollutants. Depletion of the rain forest is responsible for 9 to 12 billion tons of CO_2 emissions in the last decade from the Amazon region alone.[67]

human (and animal) welfare

Last, the animal industry isn't just tough on the animals. Yes, the lives and deaths of farm animals are often horrifyingly brutal, both physically and psychologically, but the lives of the workers on these farms (most of whom are underpaid illegal immigrants) are terrible, too. For example, in 2005, the Human Rights Watch found that "meat and poultry industry

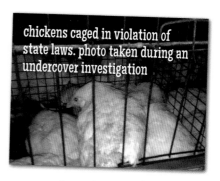

chickens caged in violation of state laws. photo taken during an undercover investigation

employers set up the workplaces and practices that create these dangers, but they treat the resulting mayhem as a normal, natural part of the production process, not as what it is—repeated violations of international human rights standards."[68]

The single largest factor contributing to worker injuries is line speed. Workers are pressured to kill more animals in less time, sometimes being paid by piece. Most meat and poultry facilities also operate nearly *twenty-four hours a day, seven days a week*. As one worker stated, "The line is so fast there is no time to sharpen the knife. The knife gets dull and you have to cut harder. That's when it really starts to hurt, and that's when you cut yourself."[69] The long hours and repetitive stress cause workers to suffer chronic pains in their hands, wrists, arms, shoulders, and back.

According to the U.S. Bureau of Labor Statistics, the meatpacking industry reported 7.5 work-related injuries per 100 full-time workers, which is about 21 percent higher than the overall food manufacturing industry and 50 percent higher than the manufacturing industry as a whole.[70] Some experts believe these numbers are actually much higher, saying many immigrants don't come forward about injuries out of fear of deportation or losing their job. (Most workers take these low-paying, backbreaking jobs out of desperation to feed their families.)

If that's not bad enough, factory farmworkers also routinely inhale hazardous levels of ammonia and hydrogen sulfide gases and particulate matter, all of which are known to cause severe health complications.[71]

In a *New York Times* interview about conditions on a foie gras farm, duck feeder Maura Gonzales Rusas described her workday: force-feeding 350 ducks three times a day, totaling more than a thousand feedings per day. Ms. Gonzales often gets only four hours of sleep per night, between her 10 p.m. to 1 a.m. shift and her 6 to 9 a.m. shift (plus she has a third shift in the afternoon). These feedings are also continuous for thirty days, at which time the ducks are slaughtered. Workers in other animal industries, such as cow milkers, have similar schedules.[72]

Approximately 99 percent of all animal products consumed in the United States come from animals raised in factory farms. When you buy meat, fish, dairy, and eggs, you're supporting this hazardous industry that exploits both humans and the animals.[73]

To learn more information on the effects of animal farming and global depletion, see the resources under Animal Welfare in the Appendix, "Learn More about Plant-Based Living."

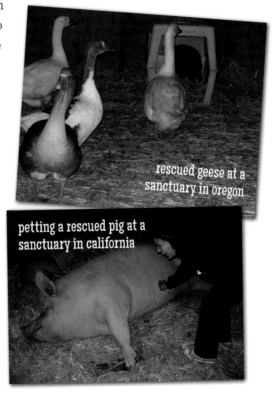

rescued geese at a sanctuary in oregon

petting a rescued pig at a sanctuary in california

ELONDRA: COLLEGE STUDENT SPREADING THE PLANT-BASED DIET ON CAMPUS
march 2012

HH: What made you adopt a plant-based (vegan) diet?

My parents became vegan about two years ago and I immediately saw a major change in their health, attitude, and weight. Many people in my family are obese and suffer many health issues, which has always frightened me, because I don't want to have the same issues.

HH: Did they talk to you about their new lifestyle? How did you learn about it?

My mom and dad persuaded me to watch *Forks Over Knives* in September 2011, and I instantly changed my diet. Ever since then, I have constantly been switching between being vegan and vegetarian. The longest I was able to hold a plant-based (vegan) diet was for five months straight. Other than that, I stuck with vegetarianism. I am still aiming toward becoming 100 percent vegan for the rest of my life.

HH: Do you find it difficult to maintain a plant-based diet while at college?

Even though a plant-based diet makes me feel so much better in so many ways, it is still a constant challenge as a student. The hardest part is the free food.

HH: How do you cope?

I have to tell myself every day that my health is worth it. I'm not perfect with my diet, but I have learned how to eliminate the common unhealthy food choices that many college students make.

On another note, my mom is the person I like to talk to when I struggle with being vegan. I feel like all I need to do is look at her in order to be encouraged to develop a plant-based diet. She has such healthy skin and hair, as well as no longer being

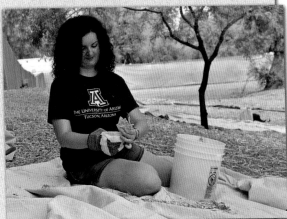

obese. Her energy is better than the average energy of somebody my age (early twenties)! Isn't that saying something? *The Happy Herbivore Cookbook* has definitely been one of my favorite cookbooks to use with my mom whenever I come back home from college!

HH: How have you overcome these challenges?

An example would be that everything in my kitchen is vegan. This forces me to cook with vegan-friendly foods all the time. A step such as this has already made a huge change in my diet. Now, if I ever have an urge to eat something unhealthy and non-plant-based, it forces me to spend money that I don't really have. In other words, it forces me to think about if the unhealthy choice is worth it for me.

HH: What other steps have you taken to making a plant-based diet easier on campus?

While on the journey of being vegan and living on campus, I also discovered that being vegan on a university's meal plan is not so simple. Along with some help from other "foodie" friends, we ended up getting a couple of other students together and

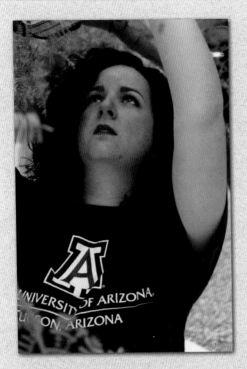

university as the Sustainable Food Production Intern. I organized a group of volunteers to help me harvest mesquite trees over the summer and collect the mesquite pods. Mesquite pods can be milled down into very sweet gluten-free pastry flour. The university's kitchen staff used the flour to prepare vegan gluten-free pastries. The mesquite harvesting on my campus is now a part of a project called LEAF (Linking Edible Arizona Forests), which is through the University of Arizona Campus Arboretum. I am serving as a student intern to help continue this project throughout the campus and local communities. I have decided to use my research and work for this project as a part of my senior capstone for the Sustainable Built Environments degree.

UPDATE (summer 2014):

I graduated from my university this spring! I graduated with a BS in Sustainable Built Environments through the College of Architecture in Planning, and Landscape Architecture at the University of Arizona. The school asked me to speak at my graduation in front of nearly a thousand people to represent my class of Sustainable Built Environments.

Now that I have graduated, I am eager to focus on becoming 100 percent vegan!

created a club called the Food Committee. The Food Committee still exists today and continues to make small changes on campus and educate students about sustainable diets.

HH: Wow! Incredible! Talk about taking the initiative! What's going on with the Food Committee now?

The Food Committee is still in the process of making a change within my university's food options. The group continues to get many campus employees by their side to help the Food Committee get to this goal. The Food Committee has also opened up many other opportunities for me.

HH: What kind of opportunities?

I worked for the Office of Sustainability at my

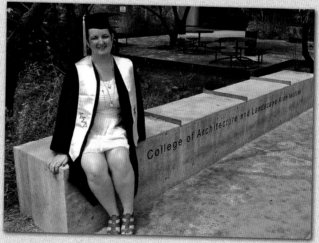

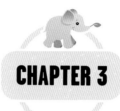

CHAPTER 3

what to expect

"Only one person in the world
can defeat you. That is yourself!"

—UNKNOWN—

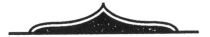

This may shock you, but I believe the single most significant decision I can make on a day-to-day basis is my choice of attitude. It is more important than my past, my education, my bankroll, my successes or failures, fame or pain, what other people think of me or say about me, my circumstances, or my position. Attitude is that "single string" that keeps me going or cripples my progress. It alone fuels my fire or assaults my hope. When my attitudes are right, there's no barrier too high, no valley too deep, no dream too extreme, no challenge too great for me.

—CHARLES R. SWINDOLL, *MAN TO MAN*—

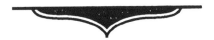

One thing being plant-based has taught me about living life is that *attitude is everything*. I love this quote by Charles R. Swindoll: "Words can never adequately convey the incredible impact our attitude is toward life. The longer I live the more convinced I become that life is 10 percent what happens to us and 90 percent how we respond to it."

It didn't take me long to realize that if I went into a meal thinking I would enjoy it, I did, and that the opposite was just as true: If I thought I was going to be disappointed or wouldn't like something, I usually didn't, because I'd made my mind up and closed myself off to the possibility before I sat down.

The more positive and optimistic I was about my new diet and lifestyle, the more I enjoyed it and tried new things with open curiosity. If you expect to have a good experience, chances are you'll have a good experience!

Along those same lines, I found it helpful not to dwell on the perceived negatives. For example, if the plant-based diet starts feeling too limited, focus on all the foods you *can* have. Start writing a list of all the fruits, vegetables, grains, and beans you can eat. Without fail, any time I task a frustrated client with completing this exercise, they tire of writing long before coming anywhere close to completing the list.

And I get it: When all you know is meat and potatoes and you take away the meat, it's easy to get caught up in staring at the potatoes. But your diet is so much more than potatoes!

I eat a much wider variety of foods now as a plant-eater than I ever did as an omnivore or vegetarian. I enjoy cuisines (Ethiopian, Indian, Thai, just to name a few) and ingredients I never would have tried before. My palate is also more refined: Foods that once seemed bland to me now have complex flavors. Foods I hated, like mushrooms, mustard, and hot spices, I now love and seek out.

WHERE'S THE BEEF?

here's a tip from my husband: Stop looking for meat on your plate. If you've eaten a Western diet until now, it's likely that meat has always been the centerpiece of the meal, with vegetables as garnish on the side. Don't let this old thinking color your new eating habits. A plate full of fruits, vegetables, grains, and beans *is* a meal. Think of these foods as the main course and remind yourself that your plate doesn't have to revolve around or even contain meat to be a meal.

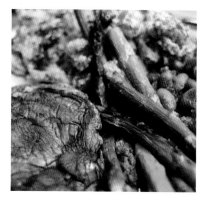

My story is not unique. I've heard it a hundred times over from others. A new world opens up to you when you go plant-based! You'll see!

Most importantly, remind yourself that it's not that you *can't* have something, but that you *choose* not to. This slight adjustment in thinking is very powerful! Keep a positive attitude. Have great expectations. Be optimistic! Smile! You'll love your new diet and lifestyle.

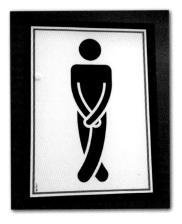

Your body may need some time to adjust to your new diet and lifestyle. You may experience withdrawal symptoms to food addictions (see "Food Addictions," chapter six) or your digestive system might have a few . . . *hiccups* (that's my cutesy way of saying gas and diarrhea).

Be patient—your body will adjust to the change over time. How much time is different for everyone; generally, it can take anywhere from a couple of days to several weeks.

flatulence

Toot! Toot! An increase in gas is a common side effect when you first switch to a plant-based diet, due to increased fiber and carbohydrate consumption.

Long process short, whatever food your body is not able to digest or absorb before it reaches the large intestine produces gas as it's broken down in the large intestine. Over time, your body will adjust to the increase in fiber and carbohydrates in your diet, and more of it will be broken down in the small intestine, meaning less undigested food will make its way to the large intestine where gas is created.

Some plant foods, however, will produce gas no matter how long you've been eating them. Beans, lentils, split peas, broccoli, cauliflower, brussels sprouts, cabbage, and asparagus cause most people to have gas. To reduce the amount of gas these foods produce, cook them well and chew them to a cream (to the consistency of mush). Soaking legumes overnight before cooking can also reduce the gas they produce.

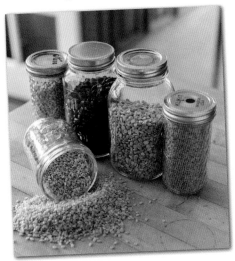

Greasy or processed foods and soy products can also cause gas. Processed soy foods—those containing soy protein isolates, such as imitation meats—tend to cause gas in most people, whereas whole forms of soy (e.g., edamame, tempeh, and tofu) are generally milder on the digestive system. Fiber supplements, including foods enriched with extra fiber like commercial cereals, may also cause gas.

Gas can also be caused by swallowing air (aerophagia), so chew your food well and swallow slowly.

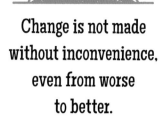

Change is not made without inconvenience, even from worse to better.

−RICHARD HOOKER−

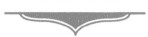

elimination

Constipation is commonly caused by inadequate fiber, so if you've previously had a diet that was low in fiber (animal-based foods contain zero fiber and most processed foods are also inadequate), you may find after switching to a plant-based diet that you're eliminating with increased frequency.

Most commercial supplements for gas (like Beano) are encased in a gelatin capsule or contain milk products. However, Bean-zyme, available at most health shops and on Amazon, is plant-based and vegan.

An enzyme in papaya has also been shown to help with gas and bloating. You can eat the fruit directly, or take papaya enzyme pills or chews (sold at drugstores). Popular herbal remedies include ginger, ginger tea, and apple cider vinegar mixed with water. Coffee or hot sauce can also stimulate bowel movements in some people.

Constipation (or the reverse) may also be caused by food sensitivities or intolerances. Keeping a food journal can help you identify any sensitivities you might have. Once you know your triggers, you can better avoid them. *For more information on food allergies, food sensitivities, and treatment, see "Sensitivities and Food Allergies" later in this chapter.*

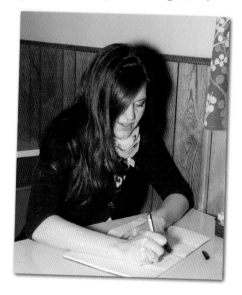

a new (and improved) normal

Many of my clients, after adopting a plant-based diet, realize discomforts they thought were normal are not. After decades of suffering and embarrassment they find they don't have to experience gas, constipation, bloating, diarrhea, or heartburn. My clients were delighted to discover they no longer had to pop pills before and after eating to avoid pain. It all went away when they started eating plant foods, often at the next meal! They often say, "I had no idea how sick I was or how truly awful I felt until I knew what it was like to feel well."

sensitivities and food allergies

People often e-mail me asking whether their new plant-based diet could make them lactose intolerant or allergic to some other food. They note how they ate the food in question (usually cheese) for years without issue and now, after a period away, they ate it again and felt terrible. What gives?

I like to think the body is giving you an affirmation that those foods are not ones you want to put inside you, and that nothing tastes as good as being healthy feels.

If a food allergy or sensitivity is presenting itself now, you probably always had this sensitivity or intolerance but didn't notice it before. If your previous diet was poor, in all likelihood there was a steady onslaught of unhealthy foods hitting your system. As a result, your body could have easily found itself overloaded with stress signals, unable to wade through the garbage and give you a specific message about a specific food.

When you clean up your diet, your body has a chance to heal, repair, and

A Warning:

Call your doctor if you experience cramping or have bloody or watery stools, chronic or persistent constipation or diarrhea, painful bloating, fever, nausea, vomiting, abdominal pain, or abdominal swelling. Additionally, if you believe you have several different food sensitivities, and bloating, gas, and/or other digestive discomforts persist, ask your doctor about leaky gut syndrome.

restore. Once it's running smoothly, you will notice each and every little hiccup with acute accuracy. It starts becoming clear just how bad "bad food" really is. Your body recognizes it for the toxic substance it is—and wants it out! Once the floor has been mopped clean, don't track the mud back in. (That said, if you're concerned about the reactions you're experiencing, you may want to consider undergoing formal allergy testing.)

Another option is going on an elimination diet. For example, eat plain potatoes for a few days until your symptoms subside. Then slowly add in different foods. Also keep in mind that some foods may be fine on their own, but cause problems when paired together. As I mentioned in chapter two, I can eat oranges and bananas by themselves with no problem, but I can't eat oranges and bananas together. If you have questions or concerns about starting an elimination diet, talk to your doctor.

women and the plant-based diet

It is perfectly safe for women to be plant-based or to transition to a plant-based diet at any stage of life, including during menopause and pregnancy (a plant-based diet can help make both better!), and while breast-feeding. There's also new evidence that a plant-based diet can boost fertility!

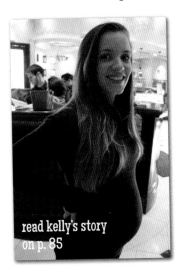

read kelly's story
on p. 85

pregnancy and breast-feeding nutrition

People often ask me if you can be plant-based when you're pregnant, trying to get pregnant, or breast-feeding. The answer is yes, absolutely! As Dr. McDougall explains, "Reproduction of the species is the primary biologic purpose of a woman. For the human being, just like all other animals, the proper source of these nutrients remains the same whether pregnant or not."[1]

Pregnancy and breast-feeding *do* place increased nutritional demands on the mother, but a plant-based diet can reasonably meet these demands, and in some cases, make it easier for mama to reach her nutritional needs.

Plants can also make for a more pleasant pregnancy. In our modern society, pregnancy has practically become synonymous with sickness and misery, but carrying a *bebe* doesn't have to be the irritable, gassy, constipated, fat, and fatigued hormonal nightmare that's billed as "normal." You *can* be a glowing goddess! Ditch the "normal" diet, hop on the plant-based highway, and follow these guidelines during pregnancy.

PROTEIN DURING PREGNANCY

The dietary reference intake (DRI) for protein during pregnancy and breast-feeding is 71 grams per day, which is about 25 grams higher than pre-pregnancy.[2] Most plant-based mamas and mamas-to-be have no problem meeting this demand. (To calculate your intake, use any free online diet program to track your food. It'll give you a breakdown of calories, carbohydrates, fats, and protein grams consumed per day.)

If you have trouble getting to 71 grams, focus on eating more high-protein plant foods like beans, lentils, leafy greens, soy products, nuts, seeds, quinoa, and other grains. Although unprocessed whole foods are always the best choice, if you find it's difficult for you to eat whole foods (or any food) due to morning sickness, consider sipping vegan protein shakes made from soy, rice, or hemp protein powders. A few of my pregnant clients had success making chocolate or fruit-flavored shakes and smoothies with vegan protein powders, vegan yogurts or ice creams, frozen bananas, and cocoa or other fruits for flavoring, like straw-berry or mango. You can also add fresh or frozen spinach, peas, nuts or nut butters, or silken (soft) tofu to your smoothies for extra protein.

CALCIUM DURING PREGNANCY

The DRI for calcium is 1,000 milligrams daily for women ages nineteen to fifty.[3] Many plant foods are rich sources of calcium (*see the table Plant-Based Sources of Essential Vitamins and Minerals),* and calcium absorption from plant foods is often superior to that of dairy products. Pregnant women who include calcium-rich plant foods in their daily diet should easily meet their needs.

ESSENTIAL FATTY ACIDS DURING PREGNANCY

The Institute of Medicine has set the adequate intake for alpha-linolenic acid (ALA) at 1.4 grams per day for women ages nineteen to fifty during pregnancy. Flaxseed is the most concentrated source of ALA, but ALA is also found in walnuts and soybeans. ALA also converts in the body into omega-3 fatty acids DHA and EPA. If you remain concerned about getting adequate DHA during pregnancy, you might consider Neuromins, microalgae supplements.[4] (*See the Fatty Acids (or Fish-Oil) Myth for more information on fatty acids.*)

IRON DURING PREGNANCY

Iron-deficiency anemia is not uncommon during pregnancy, whether the mother is plant-based or omnivore. Iron supplements or prenatal vitamins containing iron are often prescribed for women on any kind of diet.[5] Plant-based mamas should strive to eat iron-rich plant foods like greens, whole grains, tofu, and beans during pregnancy. (*See the Plant-Based Sources of Essential Vitamins and Minerals on page 35 for a list of iron-rich foods.*) It's interesting to note that pairing iron-rich foods with foods containing vitamin C increases iron absorption, but pairing iron-rich foods with high-calcium foods *decreases* iron absorption.[6]

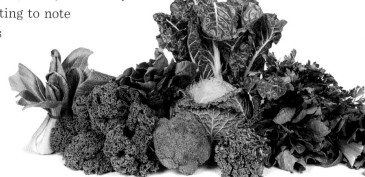

FOLATE AND FOLIC ACID DURING PREGNANCY

Plant-based diets tend to be naturally high in folate, which is needed in early pregnancy. Folate is the naturally occurring form of vitamin B_9. Greens, beans, vegetables, mushrooms, oranges, and beans are high in folate. Folic acid, on the other hand, is the synthetic form of this vitamin. Many cereals, flours, and pastas are enriched or fortified with folic acid.

To be on the safe side, women capable of becoming pregnant should take a supplement or consume fortified foods that provide 400 micrograms of folate per day. Pregnant women need 600 to 800 micrograms of folate per day.[7]

Interestingly, folic acid is more absorbent than folate. For example, 60 micrograms of folic acid has the same bioavailability as 100 micrograms of folate.[8]

Mixed research exists on whether excessive folic acid increases cancer risk, however, so stick to whole foods with folate as much as possible.

VITAMIN B_{12} DURING PREGNANCY

The recommended dose of vitamin B_{12} for pregnant women ages nineteen to fifty is 2.6 micrograms per day, a slight increase from 2.4 micrograms per day for nonpregnant women. While many foods are fortified with B_{12}, it is prudent to take a vitamin B_{12} supplement during pregnancy for added precaution.[9] (*See "The Vitamin B_{12} Myth" in chapter one for more information.*)

ZINC DURING PREGNANCY

Pregnant plant-based women may have higher zinc needs because of lower absorption of zinc on a plant-based diet. Legumes, nuts, whole grains, and cereals are rich sources of zinc. You can also increase zinc absorption by including sprouted grains, beans, seeds, and yeast-raised breads into your diet, by soaking and cooking legumes, and by combining zinc sources with acidic ingredients such as lemon juice or tomato sauce.[10] Zinc is also often included in prenatal vitamins.

VITAMIN D DURING PREGNANCY

Vitamin D, also called the sunshine vitamin, is important to both mother and baby. Although vitamin D needs do not increase during pregnancy, expectant and nursing mothers should take extra care to ensure they are getting enough vitamin D. Talk to your doctor about supplements and ask to have your levels tested.

women and fertility

Too little research has been done on fertility and diet, but the research we do have suggests that endometriosis, polycystic ovary syndrome (PCOS), and a number of other conditions that may affect fertility are related to diet and may be treated or alleviated with a plant-based diet.

Dr. McDougall explains, "A diet low in fat and high in fibrous carbohydrates...helps reverse insulin resistance, which affects 50 percent to 70 percent of women with PCOS."[11]

He also adds, "Studies of populations of women show the risk of developing endometriosis is much higher with the consumption of red meat and beef, and much lower with the consumption of vegetables and fruits. A similar dietary connection is found with other diseases of the female reproductive organs, including uterine fibroids, ovarian cysts, and cancers of the uterus (endometrium) and ovary."[12]

Results from the 2007 Nurses' Health Study—the largest and longest-running women's health study in the world—suggest that eating less meat and more vegetables may

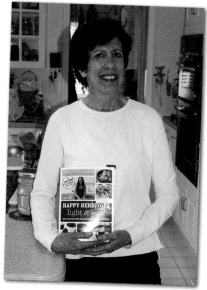

read sally's story on page 119 about how adopting a plant-based diet helped her overcome ovarian cancer!

improve fertility. The study found that women who received more protein from vegetables than from meat had significantly lower rates of infertility caused by ovulatory problems, which accounts for as much as 25 percent of all infertility cases.

This is anecdotal, but I've met several women who beat fertility issues and got pregnant after switching to a plant-based diet, even when their doctors told them

BETH: CURED FROM PCOS AND INFERTILITY

may 2013

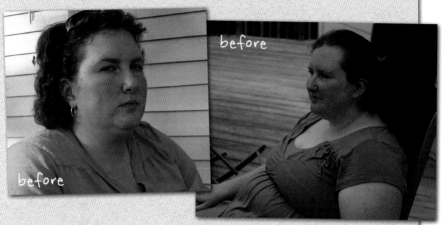

HH: I get a lot of questions about fertility and the plant-based diet. You found a correlation between the two. Can you tell us a little bit about your history and experience?

Since puberty, I have always had an irregular menstrual cycle. And when they did come, it was awful. They were very heavy, I would pass out, and I couldn't move because of debilitating cramps. I would lie on the bathroom floor in the fetal position, and nothing would help.

HH: Did you have any other medical issues or problems?

Thirteen years later, I was finally diagnosed with polycystic ovarian syndrome (PCOS). I had many other symptoms: gaining weight and trouble losing it, bad acne, facial hair, and fertility problems.

HH: Many of the women who e-mail me have PCOS and want to know if a plant-based diet can help. What have you learned? What are your experiences?

I have read a lot of information about PCOS, and everyone says it is not curable. Everyone's main goal is to manage and treat the symptoms. I have always been opposed to medicine that only treats the symptoms. I always want to know what the real problem is and treat it.

I discovered that people with PCOS often are insulin resistant, or are at a higher risk for developing insulin resistance. Because both of my parents were type 2 diabetic, I knew I had to be extra careful, since insulin resistance is a precursor to diabetes. I wanted to do whatever I could to avoid developing insulin resistance or diabetes.

HH: What did you do?

I tried changing my diet to what the doctors recommended. I cut out all white foods: white rice, potatoes, and white bread. That did not seem to help at all. I went a step further and tried the low-carb thing. That was the most miserable I have ever been.

HH: How did you find your way to a plant-based diet?

After a few months on that diet and going nowhere, I decided to watch *Forks Over Knives* on Netflix. I had no idea what it was about and hadn't heard anything about it. Everything in the film just made sense and I thought, "I am going to try this. Maybe it will work for me."

The next day, October 2, 2011, I began my new plant-based lifestyle. It was the best thing I ever did.

HH: Was the switch difficult for you?

It was rough in the beginning. I remember about two weeks into the plant-based lifestyle I got the worst headache that lasted about five days. I almost gave up. I

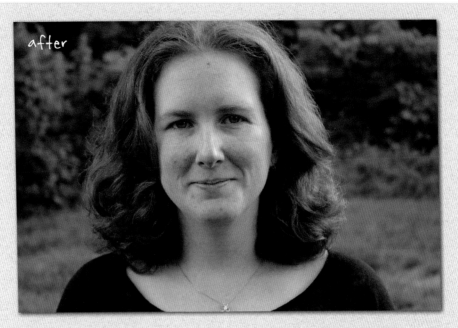

after

kept fighting through it. I think it was just my body finally beginning to detox. I felt like my eyes were sunken in, and I thought there was something wrong with me. I think it was just all the chronic inflammation in my face going away.

HH: What about the menstrual cramps and other symptoms you had? Did they go away or alleviate? When did you finally start to feel some relief after you detoxed?

Within a month, my debilitating menstrual cramps were gone. That is when I knew this was working for me. That alone was enough motivation for me to keep going on this diet. The pounds just kept flying off, too, and I kept feeling better and better.

HH: How much weight have you lost?

I have lost 72 pounds, and feel the best I ever have in my life. I know that this is a permanent lifestyle for me.

HH: Wow! That's incredible! Have you experienced any other benefits?

My other health problems went away, also. For example, my chronic constipation, which had been diagnosed as irritable bowel syndrome, was gone. I had tried everything for it in the past and nothing worked. My blood pressure was normal, and I stopped taking my blood pressure medication. My total cholesterol went from 195 to 145. My LDL went from 118 to 68.

HH: Did you quit taking any other medications?

I had been taking birth control pills to regulate my menstrual cycle, and not for pregnancy prevention. I decided to stop taking them to see if my body could now regulate itself. For four months in a row, my periods came like clockwork. Then, I became pregnant. This was a huge shocker, because my doctors had told me that due to PCOS, I would probably not be able to get pregnant on my own without medication.

UPDATE (summer 2014):

I have now lost 93 pounds. I don't need any of my old prescription medications. My total cholesterol is down to 115, LDL is down to 55, and triglyceride levels down to 119. My blood pressure now averages around 110/70. Everything is going great!

it was hopeless or extremely unlikely they'd conceive. Many have shared their stories as part of the Herbie of the Week series on HappyHerbivore.com.

contraception

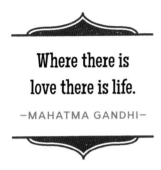

Where there is love there is life.

—MAHATMA GANDHI—

First and foremost, *I encourage every woman to talk to her doctor* about birth control options and their effectiveness in preventing pregnancy and sexually transmitted diseases and infections.

In terms of how contraceptives fit into a plant-based lifestyle . . . it's a tricky subject. Contraception is very much a personal decision, and the factors that go into that decision vary from woman to woman. What might be right for you might not be right for someone else. Ultimately, I find that at some point our diet and lifestyle becomes subject to our own interpretation and how far we're willing to go with it to appease our spiritual and moral beliefs.

For the sake of brevity, I'm going to focus only on whether contraceptives contain animal ingredients such as dairy or gelatin, and give a short overview of hormone versus non-hormone options. If you are an animal-rights vegan, other issues may be present for you, such as whether the pharmaceutical company tests on animals and if the hormones used come from plant, human, or animal sources.

HORMONE-BASED CONTRACEPTIVES

Most oral tablets (i.e., birth control pills) contain a trace amount of lactose (a dairy by-product) as an inactive ingredient. At the time of this writing, I was unable to find any U.S. brand of birth control that was 100 percent dairy-free, but I was also unable to exhaustively research every brand and generic variation available.

Other hormone-based birth control methods that are not taken orally, such as a vaginal ring or the Depo-Provera shot, do not contain lactose.

NON—HORMONE-BASED CONTRACEPTIVES

In the United States, copper IUDs (ParaGuard) are probably the most popular non-hormone contraceptive choice for women. (The only non-copper IUD options in the United States—Mirena and Skyla—release the hormone progestin.) Note that women with IUDs may or may not be able to use menstrual cups such as the Diva Cup. The information on menstrual cup manufacturer websites is conflicting. Talk to your doctor about using a menstrual cup with an IUD.

BARRIER CONTRACEPTIVES

Traditional barrier methods like condoms are typically made from synthetic latex that usually contains casein, a milk protein. Sir Richard's Condom Company, for one, makes vegan natural-latex condoms, and some companies use silicone, which is plant-based (but may have non-vegan components). Diaphragms are usually made from silicone, but may be made from latex, too.

As I said before, your method of pregnancy prevention is personal—it depends on how far you're willing to go with your plant-based lifestyle. I'm not going to send the plant-based police after you for using one method over another. Do what's right for you!

ASSOCIATED HEALTH RISKS

At the time of this writing, I was unable to find any medical studies that examine the effects, if any, of trace amounts of animal ingredients in oral contraceptives or barrier methods such as condoms on health. Perhaps the key difference there, if any, is that you actually ingest animal ingredients in oral contraceptives.

However, a 2012 study in the *New England Journal of Medicine* suggested women who take birth control pills may be at a *slightly* greater risk for heart disease and/or stroke.[13] This news spawned a flurry of e-mails from Herbies asking me for my opinion.

I'm not a doctor or medical researcher, so I can't comment much on the study's findings or conclusions. What I will say, though, is that there are risks to *any* medication we take, and if nothing else, those risks can be a great motivator to eat the healthiest diet we can.

Talk to your doctor about any potential risks your medications pose and what alternatives might be available. It's also not a bad idea to get a second opinion if you don't feel your doctor is in agreement with you about your diet, lifestyle, or goals. In addition to consulting your doctor, I encourage everyone to do their own due diligence and research online, but be sure to consult reliable sources like medical journals.[i]

---

i. The U.S. National Library of Medicine maintains a set of useful guidelines for determining if a source is reliable. "Evaluating Health Information," on its website: http://www.nlm.nih.gov/medlineplus/evaluatinghealthinformation.html.

NATURAL CONTRACEPTIVE METHODS

When I first blogged about the topic of plant-based contraception on HappyHerbivore.com, many Herbies left comments about their experiences with calendar-based methods of natural family planning. This involves monitoring your ovulation cycles and abstaining during fertility periods. Lady-Comp came widely recommended as a fertility monitor. Other methods include the Billings Ovulation Method, the Creighton Model FertilityCare System, the sympto-thermal method, and the Marquette Model. Long-term solutions such as sterilization may be another option for your family.

menstruation

Many pains and annoyances associated with the menstrual cycle are avoidable—and plant foods can help reverse "the curse"! A low-fat, plant-based diet has been shown to reduce breast tenderness and swelling in 60 to 100 percent of women afflicted with breast pain during their periods.[14]

Dr. McDougall explains, "When a woman changes to a low-fat, plant-food-based diet her reproductive hormones correct, and most troublesome female problems, like heavy menstrual bleeding, fibrocystic breast disease, and PMS are all alleviated. Her risk of future health problems such as breast and uterine cancer are also greatly reduced."[15]

Diets high in fat—particularly saturated animal fats—can cause endometrial buildup (heavier periods) while increasing the size of blood clots. The passage of these larger clots and extra buildup can cause pain during menses. This suggests that a change in diet can directly affect the pain and amount of bleeding experienced during your period.[16]

Additionally, many women have shared their experiences of how they reversed PCOS or infertility, or eliminated their womanly issues like PMS and cramping, through a plant-based diet in "A Post for the HER-bies: Menstruation and Womanly Issues" on HappyHerbivore.com.[ii]

menopause

For most women, menopause begins around ages forty-five to fifty. Some women feel fine when going through "the change," while others experience symptoms like

---

ii. See http://happyherbivore.com/2014/03/menstrual-cycle-female-issues-plant-based-diet.

hot flashes, vaginal dryness, depression, and irritability. A plant-based diet may help soothe some of these complaints. Regular aerobic exercise, such as vigorously walking for thirty minutes, is also important. Aerobic exercise can help alleviate menopausal symptoms such as hot flashes, anxiety, and depression. Low-impact exercise also decreases your risk of fracture.[17]

HOT FLASHES

Research suggests hot flashes are the result of diet. Women who eat primarily plant-based diets (e.g., Asian and Mayan women) have few instances of hot flashes, while women who regularly eat meat and dairy (e.g., American and European women) commonly complain of hot flashes during menopause. Animal-based foods also affect hormone levels, which undoubtedly contributes to menopausal symptoms.[18]

BONE LOSS

Animal proteins found in meat, dairy, and eggs contribute to bone loss and increase risk of fracture. Adequate calcium intake from plant-based sources is essential (*see "The Dairy Myth" in chapter one*). Postmenopausal women might also want to avoid salt, caffeine, and tobacco, which have been linked to accel-erated calcium loss.

men and the plant-based diet

In Western cultures, and America especially, meat consumption is heavily associated with manliness. A quick look at contemporary commercials and marketing directed at men confirms this. Nothing is more macho than eating meat—not even *football*!

A recent study in the *Journal of Consumer Research* found that "to the strong, traditional, macho, bicep flexing, all-American male, red meat is a strong, traditional, macho, bicep-flexing, all-American food." Indeed, the subjects

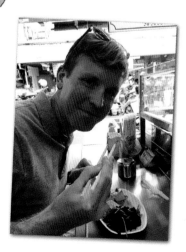

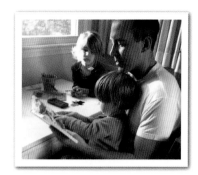

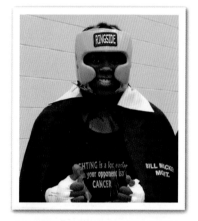

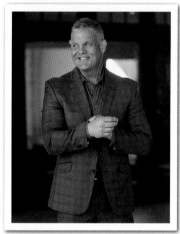

a few plant-based men featured in this book. top to bottom: tebben (see story on p. 150), cam (see story on p. 100), and david (see story on p. 28)

viewed soy meat analogues and vegetables as "weak and wimpy," and saw meat as "strong and powerful like themselves."[19] A 2012 study echoed these findings: Both men *and women* viewed eating meat as manly, and men who ate meat felt manlier after consumption. (*For more information on the relationship between meat and sexuality—and masculinity—see "Meat and Masculinity" in the Appendix, "Learn More about Plant-Based Living."*)

This meat-is-manly perception is why I think so many men have a hard time even considering the idea of not eating meat. Salads are "chick food," and being vegetarian is a *girl thing*, right?

But as my friend and former firefighter and professional triathlete Rip Esselstyn says, "Real men eat plants."

Most of the modern issues that plague men, such as erectile dysfunction and prostate cancer, have been linked to diet. The two leading causes of death among men— heart disease and cancer—have also been linked to meat consumption. A plant-based diet has been shown to lower the risks of several more major causes of death for men, such as diabetes, stroke, and kidney disease. Lest we forget: Popeye ate spinach and his rotund, burger-eating friend's name was what? Wimpy! Like Rip said, real men eat plants! (*For a list of seriously strong men who eat plants, check out "Athletes and the Plant-Based Diet" later in this chapter.*)

erectile dysfunction

Erectile dysfunction is often the first clinical sign of heart disease in men. When the body experiences atherosclerosis—the buildup of plaque (fats and cholesterol) in the arteries—smaller arteries, such as those in the penis, are usually the first to clog. (Diminished blood flow to the penis from clogged arteries makes an erection difficult.) The good news: PAD (peripheral arterial disease) and impotence (erectile dysfunction) can often be reversed with a plant-based diet.[20]

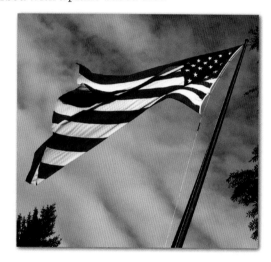

This is anecdotal, but recently I interviewed fifty plant-based men for an article, and nearly all of them reported firmer erections and a greatly improved sex life overall after switching to a plant-based diet.[21]

"Raise the Flag with a Vegan Diet," a video by Forks Over Knives (which produced the 2011 documentary of the same name), provides a good overview of the relationship between a plant-based diet and sexual virility.[22]

prostate problems

Several studies have linked red meat, processed meats, and dairy products with prostate cancer or an increased risk of prostate cancer.[23] Perhaps the most convincing evidence is a 1958 report confirming by autopsy that there were only eighteen deaths from prostate cancer in the *entire* nation of Japan that year. (In 1958 Japanese men ate a predominately plant-based diet.)[24]

There is also evidence that an enlarged prostate is linked to the consumption of meat and dairy as well: "Long-term overstimulation of the prostate gland with male hormones, such as testosterone, is believed to be the cause of benign prostate enlargement. Higher testosterone levels are found in men who eat foods rich in fats. Malignant enlargement, caused by cancer cells, is believed to be provoked by the same agencies."[25]

BRIAN: PLANT-STRONG CANCER SURVIVOR

september 2013

HH: When did you take the plant-based plunge?

I became vegan in January 2012. I have had two or three slip meals since but other than that have maintained a plant-based diet.

HH: What motivated you to adopt a plant-based diet?

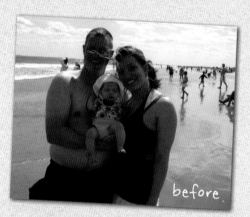

before

The first motivation was my wife, Kelly. She became vegan in August 2011. Originally, she was going to slowly transition over the final four months of 2011, but then she read *The Kind Diet*, and that was it. She was vegan the next day. At that point, she cooked her (vegan) meals and I would eat those along with some chicken, fish, and steak. After all, I needed my protein! Toward the end of the year, I watched *Forks Over Knives* and then I knew it was time for me to make the switch.

The second motivation was my health. In December 2008, I was diagnosed with colon cancer. It was rather surprising considering that I was only thirty-three. I had surgery, chemo, and radiation.

My surgeon talked to me about the role that my diet could have played in the development of my cancer. He explained

how other cultures did not experience colon cancer at the same rate as those who eat a Western diet. I had filed that in the back of my head. Then once Kelly went vegan, I knew it was time to start treating my body better.

The third motivation was that I was fat. I saw how quickly and easily my wife was dropping weight without working out or restricting calories, and I wanted in!

HH: Anytime I'm talking to Herbies, the subject of other men, specifically teasing and questioning manhood, comes up. Have you received any teasing or flak from other men?

Yes. I just am very forthright in my opinions. Heck, I am from New York, and it's the only way I know how to be. I believe in honoring my body, the planet, and animals, and I will defend my dietary choices. If I felt that someone was judging me (not eating "manly foods"), I would probably remind them that meat leads to impotence.

HH: You crack me up! Any advice for others looking to make the switch?

Just do it. I just think people think that it is so much harder than it really is. Also if you slip up . . . SO WHAT? Just start fresh right away and keep

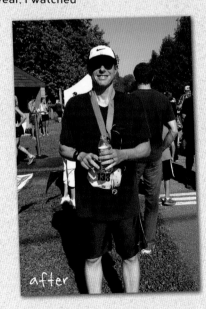

after

going. And you will get plenty of protein. Go talk to elephants and gorillas if that worries you at all.

I feel better. I lost 50 pounds and I have more energy.

KELLY (brian's wife):

I couldn't be more proud of Brian and I would like to brag on him just a bit more.

When Brian and I met, he was in New York working in finance, and was very successful but also feeling unfulfilled and unsatisfied. After some encouragement to follow his heart and passion, he quit finance and has never looked back! And after some time off and some soul-searching, he knew what I and everyone else already knew, that he was meant to *help* people, which began his journey into nursing.

A man as intelligent and driven as Brian could easily have gone to medical school, but he really wanted to go into nursing. It's an "in the trenches" way of really making a difference in people's health care.

Right around Christmas of 2008 he was diagnosed with stage 3 colon cancer. We were shocked to say the least. I was pregnant with our first child, and we were scared.

Our journey to plant-hood came from the passing mention of a doctor who said that colon cancer simply doesn't exist where they don't eat red meat.

This concept floored me. From that day forward I knew that diet and health were closely linked, and we quit red meat then and there. We stayed in this holding pattern for quite a while, until I found *The Kind Diet* and then T. Colin Campbell's books on health and dieting.

I knew Brian would never go for it, so I changed my own diet that day in August 2011 and he quietly stood by as I relearned how to cook all over again. Truth be told, I think he liked all the new foods and flavors, but he remained skeptical until New Year's Eve of 2011. That was the day he watched *Forks Over Knives*.

Brian shook his head, stopped at the all-you-can-eat sushi on the way to work,

and with every bite thereafter, he committed himself to plant eating. Yes, there has been the odd meal or bite here and there that aren't plant-based, but he is clearly thriving!

His before and after pictures speak for themselves, but it's worth mentioning that now, four years after cancer, Brian looks ten years younger, is a full-time student (with incredible grades), working weekends, and just ran his first half-marathon (2:00:13)! There is nothing he cannot do! His energy is that of a teenager.

People cannot believe he's fast closing in on forty! He inspires me daily by all that he does and has done, but maybe most important of all, every scan, test, blood draw poke, or prod he's had postcancer has been not just clean, but astonishingly clean! I have NO DOUBT he will live to be a hundred! (And probably just as active and spunky then as he is now.)

Lindsay's recipes have helped Brian regain his health and kept him from reaching for a bacon, egg, and cheese sandwich. They have helped save my husband's life. Thank you, Lindsay, I'm eternally indebted to you.

UPDATE (fall 2014):

I have since graduated nursing school (this past spring), and Kelly and I also welcomed a second child this summer.

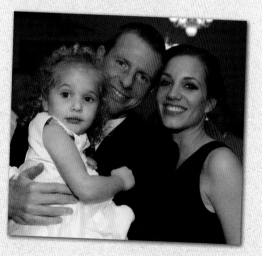

male pattern baldness

Dr. Masumi Inaba, author of *Can Human Hair Grow Again? Baldness: New Steps Toward Prevention and Cure* (Azabu Shokan, 1985), found a direct correlation between increased levels of animal fats eaten by men in Japan and an increased incidence of male pattern baldness in Japanese men. Before World War II, almost every Japanese man in Japan had a full head of hair. After moving to Hawaii or California, or changing their diet in Japan, a number of Japanese men become bald—just as some white and black American men. Dr. Inaba proposed that the loss of hair is the result of increased activity of sebaceous glands in the scalp, caused by the overstimulation of these glands by testosterone. (A diet high in animal fats results in elevated hormone levels.)

Dr. Inaba's recommended treatment was a diet low in animal fats with regular shampooing plus an oxidizing scalp treatment (to deactivate the testosterone found in scalp cells). Dr. Inaba reported mild to moderate regrowth in 30 to 53 percent of his cases.[26]

children and the plant-based diet

A plant-based diet is suitable for all stages of childhood, from birth through adolescence and into adulthood. The best way to ensure your child is hitting growth benchmarks is to make sure he or she is getting enough calories. The trouble is that kids have high caloric needs but tiny tummies, so they often feel full

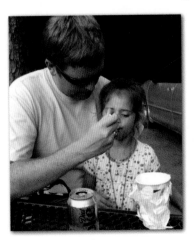

before they've consumed enough. And plant foods can be particularly problematic because they tend to contain lots of water and fiber, which fills kids up fast but on too few calories.

Concentrated calorie sources like dried fruits, nuts, seeds, grains, avocados, vegan yogurt, coconut milk, smoothies, and vegan muffins are good choices for children. It also helps to keep plenty of snacks around so your kiddo is constantly munching. Dry, whole-grain cereals and peanut butter on crackers are a couple of great, calorie-packed snacks for kids.

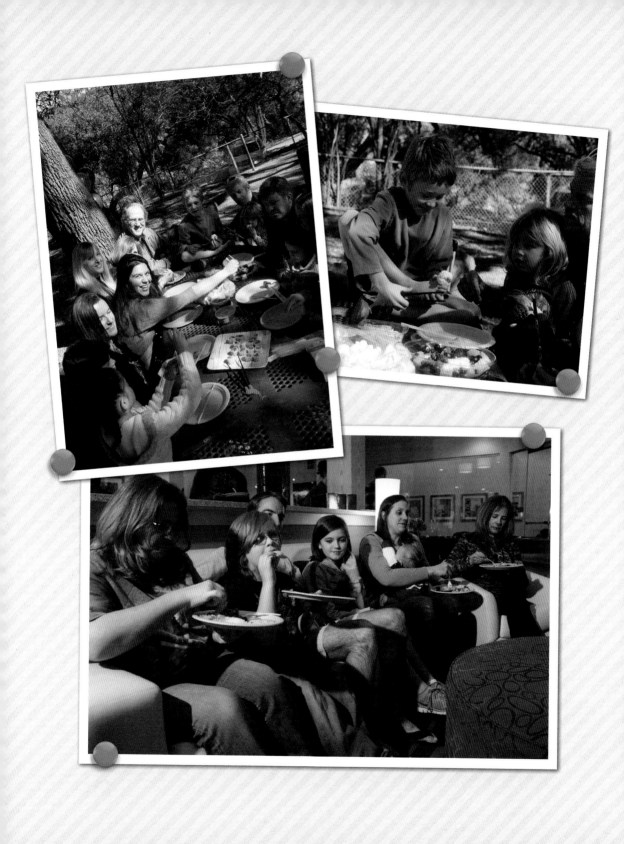

MICHELLE: REMARKABLE CHANGES IN KIDS ON A PLANT-BASED LIFESTYLE

september 2013

HH: What made your family switch to a plant-based diet?

About eleven months ago, my husband found out he had high blood pressure. He was only thirty and we knew we needed to make some changes to our diet. We weren't exactly sure what changes needed to be made. I talked with some friends about how we could get his blood pressure down. One friend suggested trying a Paleo diet. We thought we would give that a try. About a month into it, we just didn't feel that it was right for us.

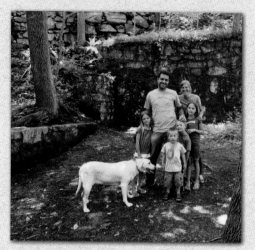

We couldn't understand how a diet full of meat, nuts, and oil was going to bring his blood pressure down. Another friend told me I should watch *Forks Over Knives*. One night in June 2012, my husband and I sat down and watched it. That night after finishing the documentary, we knew that we needed to switch our family of six to a plant-based diet. The next day, I threw out everything we had containing meat and dairy.

HH: Has your family experienced any benefits of a plant-based diet?

Now, ten months later, my husband's blood pressure is in normal limits. We have also seen so many wonderful changes in our children. This diet isn't just for people with high blood pressure, high cholesterol, diabetes, trying to lose weight, and so forth. Children really benefit and adapt very well.

HH: What are some of the positive changes you've seen in your children?

My two boys have had trouble with ear infections, swollen tonsils, and adenoids since they were six months old. They have had to have two sets of tubes in their ears, as well as their tonsils and adenoids removed. Since following a plant-based diet, they have not had one ear infection. I took them

to the ear, nose, and throat doctor for a checkup in December 2012 and she said, "I have never seen these boys so clear. Their tubes have fallen out and they look better than I have ever seen them." She added, "If they look this good in the winter, I don't need to see them any longer." That was awesome news.

HH: That's incredible! I had horrible earaches as a kid, too. I've heard from a number of parents that nixing dairy does wonders for kiddos with ear, nose, and throat problems. Have there been any other benefits with the kids?

We found out that one of my sons has a milk allergy. It was causing him to be sick with ear infections, runny nose, and eczema all over his face. We didn't even know it was dairy that was causing all of these problems until we cut it out.

HH: How did you uncover this hidden allergy?

In February 2013, I let my kids have an ice cream sundae. Within an hour, this child that we now know has an allergy felt so sick, with a runny nose and a thick rash all over his face and neck. His throat was itching and he felt like it was closing up. I gave him

Benadryl and it resolved. I think it had been so long since he had dairy that his body didn't know how to handle it.

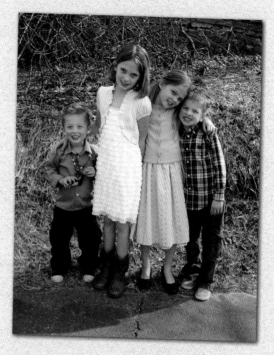

HH: Many parents, plant-based or omnivore, worry about their kids not getting all the vitamins they need. How are your kids doing on a plant-based diet?

I had my kids' vitamin and hemoglobin levels checked in March 2013. Their levels were higher than they had ever been. One of my children's hemoglobin level is usually around 10. It was 14.2 at the testing. I just can't tell enough people how many wonderful things can come out of changing to a plant-based diet.

HH: What about you, Michelle? Have you experienced any benefits?

I used to have to take a nap every day. I now have so much energy, I wouldn't even be able to fall asleep if I tried to nap.

HH: Do your kids help out in the kitchen? How have they taken to the plant-based lifestyle?

My kids now have unprompted competitions over which one of them can make the best salad using kale and collard greens topped with the 3-2-1 Dressing from *The Engine 2 Diet*. They fight over who gets to lick the bottom of the popcorn bowl clean of nutritional yeast! They are choosing to make fruit salad for dessert over eating Easter candy.

HH: When you're the first of your peers to go plant-based, it can feel rather isolating. How have you coped?

I have started a private group on Facebook that has been a wonderful way for me to encourage others to eat a plant-based diet and share all the information I am learning. I think to stay plant-strong, it really helps to have a group of like-minded people for support.

HH: Is there anything else that helps keep you and your family plant-based?

We love the Happy Herbivore meal plans. They make my life so much easier. I have been saving time and money by using them. I also love that when using the meal plan, I feel like I can eat a lot of food and maintain my current ideal weight. I never feel hungry.

My family has committed to being plant-strong for life. I am excited to continue to learn daily and encourage others to make changes by cutting meat and dairy out of their diets.

Here are some of the foods my mother made for me as well as other ideas from Herbie parents.

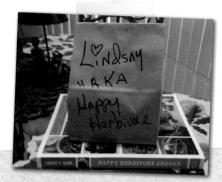

school lunch

- ☐ soups in Thermos
- ☐ PB&J (or PB & banana) sandwiches [27]
- ☐ wraps or sandwiches with hummus, avocado, and/or veggies
- ☐ cucumber and vegan cream cheese sandwich
- ☐ Mock Tuna Salad sandwiches*
- ☐ Eggless Salad sandwiches*
- ☐ pizza
- ☐ "pizza" with pita, sauce, and vegan cheese
- ☐ English muffin pizzas
- ☐ tofu hot dogs
- ☐ bean burritos
- ☐ beans and rice
- ☐ nachos
- ☐ Smoky Black Bean Enchiladas*
- ☐ pasta

- ☐ pasta salad
- ☐ veggie burgers
- ☐ Quick Black Bean Burgers*
- ☐ Cheater Pad Thai*
- ☐ veggie sushi
- ☐ soba noodle salads
- ☐ broccoli and marinara
- ☐ casseroles
- ☐ Hippie Loaf*
- ☐ leftovers
- ☐ tofu and soy sauce (or other sauce)
- ☐ Spring Rolls*
- ☐ Quiche with Greens*
- ☐ Soy-Free Mac 'n' Cheese*
- ☐ Crispy Vegan "Chicken" Nuggets*
- ☐ Pancakes*
- ☐ Courtney's Waffles*
- ☐ French Toast*
- ☐ bagels with vegan cream cheese

* See recipes at happyherbivore.com/recipes.

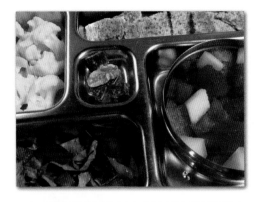

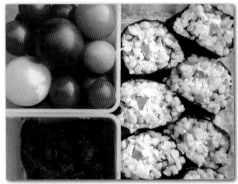

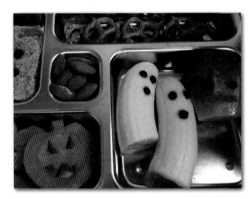

For help with transitioning kids, see chapter four, "Transitioning to a Plant-Based Lifestyle." For more transitioning tips and books and videos for parents and kids, see the Appendix, "Learn More about Plant-Based Living."

snacks

- ☐ fresh fruit
- ☐ fresh veggies (with or without dip)
- ☐ fruit and/or veggie kabobs
- ☐ soy, coconut, or almond-based yogurt (with or without granola)
- ☐ granola bars
- ☐ pretzels
- ☐ chips and salsa
- ☐ crackers (with or without peanut butter or, alternatively, sunflower seed butter)
- ☐ Zucchini Muffins
- ☐ cereal
- ☐ dried vegetables
- ☐ dried fruit
- ☐ applesauce
- ☐ popcorn
- ☐ kale chips
- ☐ trail mix
- ☐ rice cakes
- ☐ vegan cookies

drinks

- ☐ smoothies in Thermos or mason jars
  (freeze, then thaw by lunch)
- ☐ juice boxes or water boxes
- ☐ soy or almond milk

AUBREY: PLANT-BASED HIGH SCHOOL TRACK STAR
december 2013

HH: Hi, Aubrey! Tell us a little bit about yourself.

My name is Aubrey and I'm a junior in high school. I run cross country and track, and participate in Mock Trial and winter running. I also have a part-time job at a local supermarket. So, I'm pretty busy! I've been a Herbie since May 2012, which was in the middle of my track season. The week I made the change, I PRed (got a new personal record) in both of the events I run, the mile and the half-mile. I've been a Herbie ever since! The first weekend in June, I ran my first half-marathon with some of my friends! I did pretty well with a time of 1:52:04.

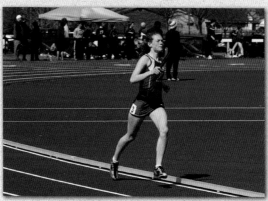

HH: Congratulations! Were you expecting an improved performance?

Since this was new for me, I was curious what my times would be like in cross country the season of my sophomore year. In my freshman year, my PR for a 5K was 23:31. My first time trial, in August (preseason), I ran faster than I ever had before with a 22:40. My final PR for sophomore year was a 21:41. I continued to improve throughout the track season with new PRs in all of my events. I ran another half-marathon right after track season, getting (coincidentally) the exact same time as the year before. That brings us to this season of cross country. After training hard and properly fueling my body, I just PRed on a 5K this Saturday with a 21:36. Fueling my body is key, especially when I'm preparing for a hard workout or a race. Those are the times I pay special attention to what I'm eating (protein, carbs, etc.). I love being a Herbie, and I have no plans of changing this in the future!

HH: That's amazing! How did you find out about the plant-based diet?

I became a vegetarian in eighth grade with influence from PETA2 (PETA's youth program), the issue then being animal rights. That was my first introduction to veganism. In my freshman year I watched *Forks Over Knives*, and that is when my mom and I dove into the plant-based diet.

HH: What's it like being plant-based in high school? How do other students and your friends react to your choice?

Being a Herbie in high school is sort of difficult sometimes, but still totally worth it. It's hard sometimes not eating pizza at parties with my friends, or passing up on cake and ice cream. But my passion for the plant-based diet makes it a lot easier to say "no" and go straight to the carrot sticks! (I *love* carrot sticks.) My friends are mostly supportive, and two of my friends are vegan as well! It makes it a LOT easier to not be the only one. Sometimes people do ask me why, and I usually say, "It's just a choice I make to keep my body as healthy as possible!" I usually don't get any arguments.

HH: As an athlete, do you notice any difference in how you feel when you are training and recovering?

I've never eaten meat while running in high school. But I did eat milk and eggs for part of my freshman year. Directly after I made the change to a plant-based diet was when I PRed in both of my track events! As training and recovery go, I have improved to be the third best varsity runner on my cross country team, so my season is going pretty great!!

HH: Do you pack a lunch for school? What kinds of foods do you like to take for lunch and snacks?

I've always packed my lunch for school, but since I've been vegan I usually pack leftovers from the night before. (That's my favorite anyway!) When there are no leftovers, I pack a lot of fresh fruit (strawberries, raspberries, blackberries, blueberries, clementines, etc.) and veggies (baby carrots, celery, romaine lettuce, peppers, etc.). I'm a big fan of Clif Bars, too, if there's no leftovers for the main course.

HH: Is your family supportive of your choice?

Yes! When I stay at my dad's house, it is a little more difficult since I am the only vegan over there, but when I am at my mom's house, it is easy, since she is vegan as well. My aunt and uncle introduced *Forks Over Knives* to the family, so they are vegan as well. This simplifies Thanksgiving and Christmas. Thanksgiving is my favorite holiday, and since almost everyone is plant-based, that makes planning the meal easy! For the family members that I have that are not Herbies, they are still very supportive of my choice.

HH: What are your favorite plant-based meals at home? Have you tried your hand at cooking?

My favorite meals are probably from *Happy Herbivore Abroad*. I LOVE all of the curries in there especially. I've done one of the Herbie cleanses (www.rebootcleanse911.com) as well (mostly for fun and because my mom was doing it), and I really liked the barley meal that was in there, as well as the chili! Yum! I made the barley meal from that cleanse myself and I love to help out in the kitchen whenever I have time! My mom is a trained chef, so I love to help her cook.

HH: Do you have any advice for others your age that are curious about making a change?

Being a Herbie is just so great. It doesn't get any better than helping the animals, the planet, and my body all at the same time! Plus it is DELICIOUS! For others thinking about making the change, do it! It's awesome. It's pretty easy and so healthy for your body. I just feel better being a Herbie. There are a lot of cookbooks out there to help and you can get your own ideas for meals from vegan restaurants or blogs or stuff like that. I would tell others to read a couple of books about the plant-based diet, so that you become educated and passionate about being a Herbie. It's a blast!!!

UPDATE (summer 2014):

I had a great track season this year! My new personal records include: 1,600 meters (1 mile), 5:44; 3,200 meters (2 miles), 12:48; and 13.1 miles (half-marathon), 1:40:18, which is about 12 minutes faster than my half-marathon time last year!

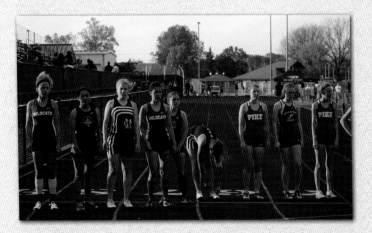

Plant-based, vegan, and vegetarian diets are taking root in professional athletics. ESPN, the *New York Times*, and the *Wall Street Journal* have all covered vegan bodybuilders and vegan and vegetarian athletes in great depth. Sports and fitness magazines like *Men's Fitness*, *Runner's World*, and *Sports Illustrated* have also published articles on plant-based diets and the benefits of eating plants for sports performance. The word is getting out!

PLANT-BASED PROFESSIONAL ATHLETES

Lizzie Armitstead
cyclist and Olympic silver medalist

Cam F. Awesome
eleven-time U.S. national champion boxer

Brendan Brazier
triathlete and two-time Canadian
Ultramarathon champion (retired)

Mac Danzig
mixed martial artist and winner of season six of
The Ultimate Fighter reality TV show (retired)

Rip Esselstyn
triathlete (retired)

Ruth Heidrich
a seventy-nine-year-old endurance runner and my
personal hero![i]

Scott Jurek
record-breaking ultramarathon runner

Billie Jean King
tennis player with thirty-nine Grand Slam titles (retired)

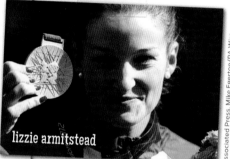
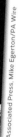

lizzie armitstead

Associated Press, Mike Egerton/PA Wire

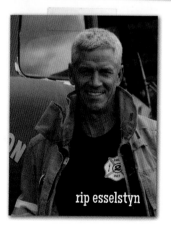

rip esselstyn

---

* Vegetarian

i. Dr. Heidrich is a breast cancer survivor and has completed the Ironman Triathlon six times, run sixty-seven marathons, accumulated more than 900 first-place trophies, and set numerous fitness records including being named one of the Ten Fittest Women in North America by *Living Fit Magazine*. She has a PhD in health management (earned in her fifties) with majors in nutrition and exercise physiology.

Carl Lewis
Olympic gold medalist

Rich Roll
endurance athlete and Ultraman World Championships top ten finisher

Dave Scott
triathlete and six-time Ironman world champion[ii]

Jake Shields
mixed martial artist

Salim Stoudamire
basketball player

Mike Tyson
boxer and world heavyweight champion 1987–1990 (retired)

Robert Parish
basketball player and Basketball Hall of Fame inductee (retired)*

Bill Pearl
bodybuilder and four-time Mr. Universe titleholder (retired)*

Billy Simmonds
bodybuilder

Herschel Walker
NFL football player and mixed martial artist (retired)*

Ricky Williams
NFL football player and Heisman Trophy winner (retired)

Serena Williams
tennis player with thirty-three Grand Slam titles and four Olympic gold medals

Venus Williams
tennis player with twenty-two Grand Slam titles and four Olympic gold medals

James Wilks
mixed martial artist (retired)

Mike Zigomanis
hockey player

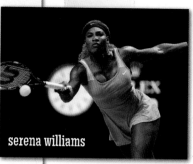

serena williams

Associated Press, Mark Baker

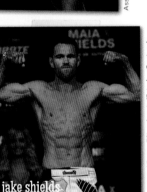

jake shields

Associated Press, Filipe Araujo/Estadao Contuedo

For information on athletic dietary needs, including protein requirements, see "The Athletes' Protein Myth" in chapter one. For more resources on vegan fitness and athletics, see the Appendix, "Learn More about Plant-Based Living."

---

ii. Scott is no longer a vegetarian, but he was vegetarian when he competed at his peak.

SHELDON: RETIRED POLICE OFFICER & PLANT-BASED KARATE CHAMPION

may 2013

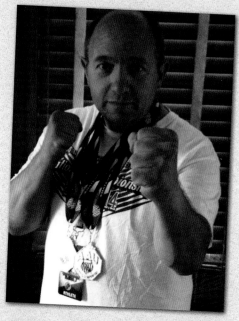

HH: I'm in total awe. I don't know where to begin! You're so impressive. Let's talk about your career as a police officer first. Tell us a little more about that.

I am a retired NYPD captain and 9/11 first responder who was decorated in the line of duty sixty times. I had one of those exciting careers that little kids dream about. Despite all the life-and-death experiences I encountered over twenty-one years, it was my diet that almost killed me.

Prior to becoming a police officer, I was an exercise physiologist. I have always maintained an extremely active lifestyle by being involved in martial arts since I was a child and also being an avid, although not very fast, runner.

HH: What was your diet and health like before adopting a plant-based diet?

Like many Americans, I ate the traditional Western diet and hid behind both the "everything in moderation" routine and "I exercise, so how bad can it get?" rationalizations.

Midway through my police career, I was diagnosed with high cholesterol and prescribed a statin. Although it hadn't sunk in yet, this was my first lesson that, as Dr. Campbell has been known to say, "you can't outwork a bad diet."

By 2004, after a routine physical, it was found out that I had a 90 percent blockage in one of my coronary arteries. I considered myself lucky to get by with just a stent. I started to make some changes, which included following the traditional "heart-healthy diet."

I retired shortly afterward, being declared disabled because of my coronary artery disease. By 2008, I found myself back in for another stent (despite my "heart-healthy diet"). I cried on the gurney as they wheeled me in. The nurse said, "Don't be afraid," and I

replied, "I'm not afraid, I'm humiliated—I used to be an exercise physiologist and this is my second stent."

HH: You eventually wound up in the hospital, but not from the stents or related complications. Tell us a little more about that.

In October 2009, I was walking my dogs when a driver ran a stop sign and plowed into me, causing me to land unconscious in a ditch with numerous broken bones and unable to walk. I was removed from the scene to a trauma unit. Strange things go through your head as they are cutting your clothes off, and I actually thought about extreme weight gain due to not being able to exercise.

I had just started working as an exercise physiologist again at a major health insurance company in a disease management program. (I wanted to turn my weaknesses into a passion and help others while also helping myself.)

By this time, I was also on a ton of other medications for blood pressure and stent-related issues. I resolved to never go back on the operating table again, and after doing my own rehab, I was walking again, then running, and doing plenty of martial arts.

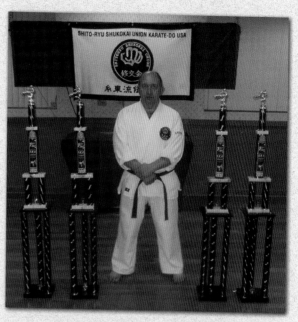

HH: After doing your own rehab? You are amazing! But I have to ask—what finally shattered your "everything in moderation . . . but I exercise" mentality? I guess what I'm asking is, how did you find your way to a plant-based diet after all this?

I struck up a friendship with a coworker and registered dietitian (RD), with whom I shared my "secret of heart disease" and sought dietary counseling as I came to grips with the fact that exercise is not a stand-alone (hey, I was a 3:11 marathoner and got stented!).

Meanwhile, another RD friend and coworker was already educating us about a whole food, plant-based diet. Then things really started to happen as I transitioned into a whole food, plant-based lifestyle.

HH: How did your family react to your dietary change?

My wife, Susan, was extraordinarily supportive, and together we explored websites like the Happy Herbivore for new ideas.

HH: What do your doctors say about all your changes?

My doctors were shocked at my changing blood pressure and cholesterol measurements. My cholesterol, once over 320, was down in the 130s. They actually started taking me off medications, something they said they would "never do."

HH: You have always been very active, fit, and athletic—but how did you get involved with martial arts and karate?

In October 2010 (the one-year anniversary of my car accident) I entered the New York State Martial Arts Championships, my first competition in over twenty years. Much to my surprise, I finished second.

In 2012, I was the number-one-ranked black belt competitor in New York State for Division 37 (age forty and over—I'm fifty-three!).

In February 2013, I won four first-place trophies at the American Karate Association Grand Nationals—making me a four-time National Champion—powered by plants!

Now, what's this nonsense about not getting enough protein from a plant-based diet?

UPDATE (winter 2014):

In January 2014 I returned to the American Karate Association Grand Nationals and won another four first-place trophies. In May 2014 I became a fifth-degree black belt, at fifty-four! I've also taken up tae kwon do (pictured with my gold and silver medals won at the 2014 AAU National Championships). I recently won the International Martial Arts Federation Karate Championships and I anticipate topping the one hundred trophy mark sometime in 2015. I've also been in the United States Martial Arts Hall of Fame as "Competitior of the Year" two years in a row.

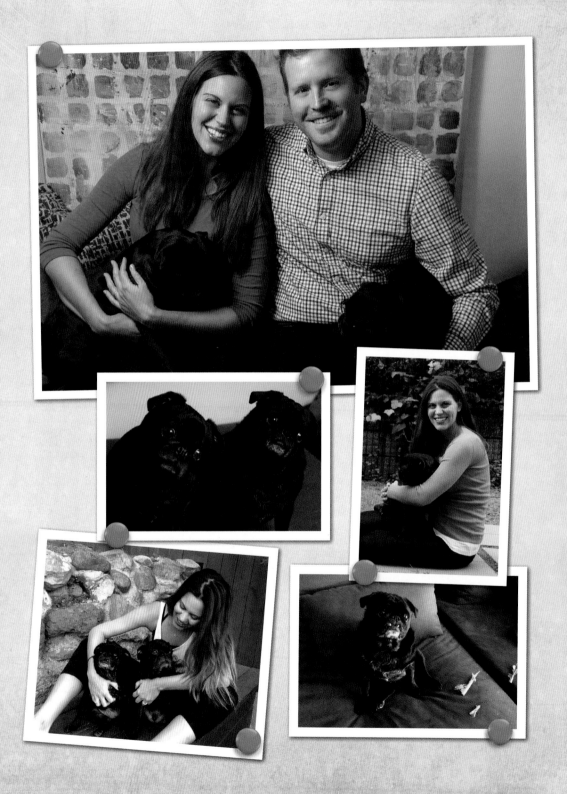

pets and the plant-based diet

What about pets? Can they be plant-based? In speaking with dozens of veterinarians, all agree most dogs can survive (and thrive!) on a plant-based diet. Cats, however, are obligate carnivores, so they must eat meat. Talk to your veterinarian before switching your furry friend to a plant-based diet, and seek their advice for how to slowly transition your pet's food.

The following companies offer a vegan or vegetarian kibble:

» AvoDerm
» Royal Canin
» Halo
» Natural Balance
» Nature's Recipe
» PetGuard
» V-Dog
» Wysong

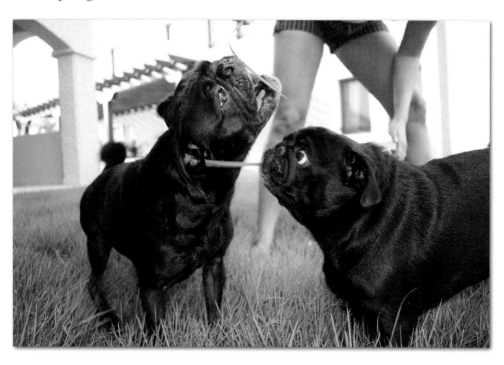

CAM: ELEVEN-TIME NATIONAL CHAMPION PLANT-BASED BOXER
march 2013

HH: What motivated you to make the switch to a plant-based diet?

Bill Mackey became my client at my boxing gym and started training for a fight. His wife, Ami, is part of the Engine 2 Team. At forty-five, Bill was 225 pounds, and due to his plant-based diet, he put on muscle and dropped fat at an amazing pace with little recovery time needed. Bill attributed his remarkable metamorphosis to his plant-based diet.

I was in a dark place and decided to change my life around, starting with my diet. The Mackeys helped me learn all about it. I have been a plant-based athlete since June 2012.

HH: Have you noticed a difference in your performance since being plant-based?

Yes, I've noticed a great difference. Before I was plant-based, I was at 260 pounds and more than 36 percent body fat, even though I was working out my hardest and boxing. I have dropped 40-plus pounds, and now I am faster in the ring. I also discovered that I had more energy to add more strength and conditioning to my regimen and became leaner, faster, and stronger. I couldn't do this before because it is impossible to outwork a bad diet!

HH: What challenges (if any) have you noticed, since plant-based eating is not too popular in sports?

One of the biggest challenges is there is never any healthy food at the gym. It's hard to find oil-free, plant-based food, but I am always prepared and bring snacks with me everywhere.

HH: Have you had to dispel the "protein is king" myth?

I get it at the gym a lot, which is funny because I am there working out and sparring constantly. When a crowd develops to watch me spar, I am pretty sure it's not due to my lack of protein.

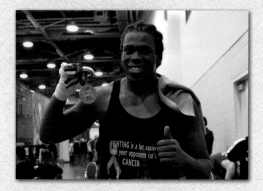

HH: Frequently, I get a lot of guys saying they're worried how other guys will perceive them, like they are less manly for not eating meat. Any thoughts or advice?

Yeah, I am guilty of making fun of a guy for eating carrots or something not so "manly." No one will say that to me, because I am a super heavyweight eleven-time national champion boxer and I dare anyone to challenge my manhood. When people think vegan, they think skinny hippie—I would like to dispel that myth.

HH: What does a meal look like for you?

A big plate of brown rice pasta with oil-free tomato sauce, onions, peppers, garlic, HH Spicy Sausage (page 150 in *The Happy Herbivore Cookbook*), and a HUGE bag of steamed spinach is one of my favorites.

UPDATE (fall 2014):

Since December 2013, I have won USA Nationals, a gold medal in the Cheo Aponte Olympic Cup, a gold medal in Poland at the Felix Stamm tournament, a gold medal in the Dominican Republic at the Independence Cup, another gold medal for the super heavyweight category at the Pan Am boxing competition in Mexico, and a fifth Ringside World Championship. I am still captain of the USA Boxing team and a proud vegan.

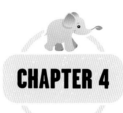

transitioning to a plant-based lifestyle

"All great change in America begins
at the dinner table."

—RONALD REAGAN—

Rip the Band-Aid off.

In theory, transitioning slowly with baby steps seems like a great idea, but in working with thousands (yes thousands!) of people transitioning to a plant-based diet, the happiest and most successful did a 180-degree turn, or close to it.

Why? You'll feel better sooner, so there will be less temptation to slide off track.

I love Pam Popper's combination lock example, explained in her book *Food Over Medicine*: "The [plant-based] diet is like a combination lock. If you have to dial four numbers to open a combination lock and you dial up three correctly, you don't get 75 percent of the results. You get nothing until you get that fourth number right. And so, we have a society filled with people who are doing 75 percent of what they need to do or 50 percent of what they need to do. They don't get 50 percent or 75 percent of the results; nothing happens until they get the whole thing right."[1]

This is anecdotal, but my parents took a lackadaisical approach for years. Yes, they had made some excellent changes like eating whole-wheat bread and pasta, adopting "meatless Monday," cooking my plant-based recipes a few times a week, and completely eliminating fast food. But they were still eating meat, dairy, eggs, processed foods, and oil, almost *every* day.

My parents would argue that, despite their chronic health issues, they were doing "pretty good." And I'd say, "Pretty good isn't good enough." Sadly, I was proven correct when my father had a mild heart attack. Initially my parents felt pretty beaten down and said things like, "Here we try to make healthy changes and your father has a heart attack anyway! Why bother?" That's when I said it was because of the changes they did make that it was a *mild* heart attack and not a fatal one. My parents quickly realized they had the gift of a second chance, went plant-based that day, and haven't wavered since. They constantly marvel at how great they feel, how much weight they've lost, and what a huge difference it makes when you go the full 100 percent. Their only complaint? They wish they had listened to me sooner. (See their full story on page 104.)

When you go "full throttle" you start to experience health benefits immediately, which solidifies your commitment and helps you keep moving in the right direction. If unhealthy foods are still coming in, they undercut your good work.

Many unhealthy foods are also addictive (*see "Food Addictions" in chapter six*), and the only way to break the addiction is to sever ties completely. And just how many times do you want to go through the pains of withdrawal and taste recalibration? Once was enough for me!

I urge you to rip off the Band-Aid. Purge the animal products, processed foods, and oil from your house. If it's around, it'll call your name. If you're living in a mixed house, create a space in the fridge, freezer, and pantry that is yours—your safe space. (*See "Mixed Households" in chapter six for tips.*)

If you feel you absolutely must take baby steps, eliminate dairy. Today. Then, next week eliminate meats—starting with fish and chicken. (Yes! Get them out first! Chicken and fish are not "healthier," despite all their fancy marketing—they have more saturated fat and cholesterol than most other popular meats!) Then cut out other meats, and eggs. The following week, cut out oil, and then work on nixing processed foods and reducing sugar and salt.

Give yourself a timeline and deadlines. Make it firm and mark it on your calendar. Otherwise you'll just get stuck and slow your progress. You can do it! If you need a foolproof guide and plan, check out my 7-Day Meal Plans (http://www.getmealplans.com)—no guesswork!

> **Yesterday is experience. Tomorrow is hope. Today is getting from one to the other as best we can.**
>
> —JOHN HENRY—

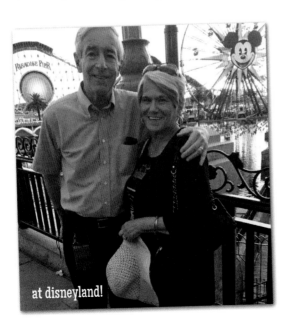
at disneyland!

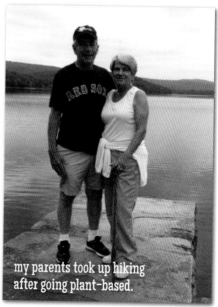
my parents took up hiking after going plant-based.

MY PARENTS: OUR DAUGHTER TALKED US INTO GOING PLANT-BASED AND WE LOVE IT

LINDSAY (september 2014):

On January 19, 2012, my dad ("Papa Herbivore") had a heart attack. Looking back, his heart attack shouldn't have come as a total surprise, but it did. In 2004, he had his first angioplasty. I had just graduated college, and had no clue about heart disease or a plant-based diet. When I asked what all this meant, my father's cardiologist was completely casual about everything, acting like the angioplasty was nothing more than a cavity filling—something that happens to everyone.

I went plant-based in late 2006, motivated by the plight of farm animals and my health. Specifically, I'd read *The China Study*, and having lost several family members to cancer, the idea of insulating myself from cancer through a plant-based diet was incredibly appealing.

Because I didn't know of anyone who had ever had a heart attack or heart surgery, heart disease was completely off my radar. For whatever reason, I thought you had to have a major cardiac emergency to have heart disease. I was completely unaware my dad had heart disease, even when he received his second stent in 2008.

From the moment I was plant-based, I encouraged my parents to adopt a similar diet, but they were resistant. They did, however, make moderate changes to their diet such as eating less fast food, switching to whole-wheat pastas and breads, and even adopting "Meatless Mondays."

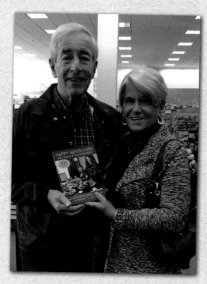

On May 29, 2011, I was on the webcam with my mom (I was living abroad at the time) when she happened to look out of the window and saw my father passed out in the grass. She ran out of the room screaming and I sat by my computer for what was easily the longest (and scariest!) twenty minutes of my life.

Several tests and specialists later, it was determined my father had a vasovagal syncope, a brief loss of consciousness.

By then I knew my father had heart disease, and I also knew the benefits of a plant-based diet for someone like him. I sent my parents a copy of *Prevent and Reverse Heart Disease* and a copy of *The China Study* for good measure. I also pushed my parents to adopt a plant-based diet, but they remained stubborn, saying, "We're doing pretty good," and I'd fire back, "But pretty good is not good enough!"

When my father had his heart attack two months later, my mother said to me, "Here we are trying to eat healthy and exercise, and your father still has a heart attack!" That's when I told her it's because they were eating healthier and exercising that he had a *mild* heart attack, and not a fatal one. "You've been given the gift of a wake-up call," I said.

In the cardiac ICU, my parents realized they weren't helpless, and that they could be in control of their lives and their health. On January 19, 2012, my Dad had a mild heart attack, and on January 20, 2012, both of my parents went plant-based.

PAPA HERBIVORE (january 2013):

Where did a year go? It has been one year since my wife and I became plant-based. Ironically, the last piece of meat I had was in the hospital after having a mild heart attack, and it was a dried-up piece of "turkey bacon." (Not my choice for a last omnivore supper.)

It's been an interesting journey. Although I know it was centered on my health condition, we both have done this together. But there are no regrets. The sacrifices were actually a lot easier than I thought they would be. I have always been a big carnivore.

Throughout this year, I can honestly say, besides the occasional urge for a big burger, I have not missed meat and have sat right next to platters of turkey, ham, meatballs, et cetera. One of the surprising things from this year is that when you tell people you are plant-based, they say, "That is so hard to do," not, "It's great that you are eating healthy." Also, when we are invited to someone's home, they are concerned about what we are going to eat. Our answer, thanks to our daughter's quote, is, "We didn't come for the food, but the company." After educating ourselves on the benefits of eating a healthy diet, we have come across many people who can't comprehend just eating plant-based. It is a mind-set; you have to want to do it for yourself, and the results speak for themselves. We feel better, have more energy, and know we can eat and still enjoy our food.

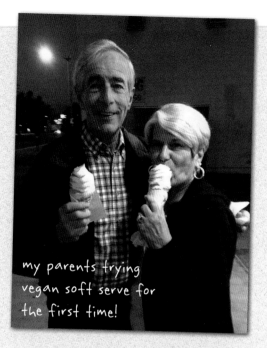

my parents trying vegan soft serve for the first time!

Another surprise is how we use so many different spices that we never would have thought to use before cooking plant-based. The combination of some of these spices and the flavors they bring out are amazing (thanks to Lindsay's wonderful recipes). One is curry—which we now love in Indian food, and let's not forget Thai food—and cayenne pepper in many recipes.

One aspect of this journey that has made it fun has been the cooking. We help each other make Lindsay's and other recipes. I am primarily the sous chef. I am trying to do more and hopefully someday will be the primary chef. But thank goodness for our daughter's easy and delicious recipes.

We have learned through the first year to stay away from most vegan processed foods. We have tried most of the "fake" meats and do not care for any of them except Boca crumbles and Spicy Chik'n patties. Other than that, we try to stay fresh and eat whole foods as much as we can and as Lindsay has guided us.

I started this journey primarily with the hope and possibility of reversing my heart disease. Only time will tell if that is happening. But other positives happened, which weren't necessarily *continued* »

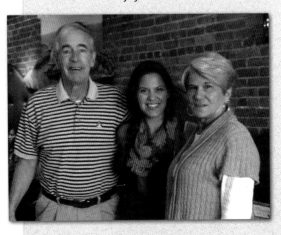

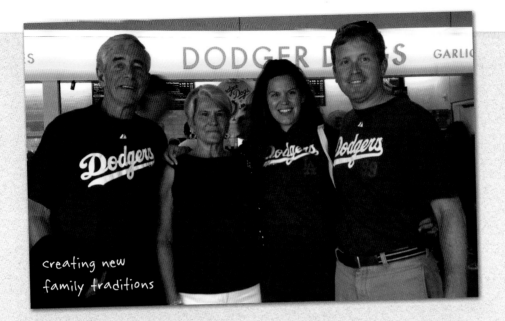

creating new
family traditions

expected. We each have lost over 20 pounds, feel so much better, have reduced our cholesterol numbers to the mid-120s, and have improved on other health stats also. What more could one ask for?

MAMA HERBIVORE (january 2013):

Our loving thanks and gratitude to our daughter Lindsay for her support, caring, and guidance. As Lindsay's mom, I personally wish that as a daughter I could have passed on to my parents some of what my daughter has taught me on eating healthier. Lindsay's grandparents would be so very proud of her today.

And finally, our special acknowledgement to all of Lindsay's fans, who have supported us and prayed for us, and particularly other Herbies, whose stories are so much more inspiring than our own.

MAMA & PAPA HERBIVORE (january 2014):

Another year has gone by, and we have now been plant-based for two years.

The year has been good to us—we are truly blessed not to have any further medical issues. Our daughter and son-in-law have a new home, and Lindsay has written another healthy and well-done cookbook.

We continue to cook from Lindsay's books, but we are now even trying to tweak some recipes on our own, using our daughter's input.

When we visit our extended family in Pennsylvania, they now respect our eating style and have even tasted and enjoyed some of the things we have made. Will our omnivore family change to plant-based? I don't know. I wish they would want to make that change, but I am grateful that maybe now they are more aware of what they are eating after being around us.

Also, as our daughter has mentioned, you can find something to eat wherever you go. We don't eat out often, but when we do, we try to find a restaurant that can accommodate us, even if it is just a salad and steamed veggies. Thai food has become one of our favorites.

Eating plant-based has now become a way of life for us. "It's just not eating, it's a lifestyle."

Our thanks again to our daughter for her guidance and support through the year, and also to the many Herbies out there for their kind words.

We will close for now by saying our New Year's resolution is to just keep on doing what we are doing and remember how good we feel.

Here are my top ten tips for making a smooth transition to the plant-based diet:

1 Take it one meal at a time. Don't worry about Thanksgiving in a few months, or a church potluck in a few weeks, or even what you're eating tomorrow. Don't get wrapped up in worries about the future. Take it a meal at a time. Focus (notice I didn't say worry!) on your next meal and don't overcomplicate things. Remember the acronym KISS—keep it simple, silly! Meals don't have to be elaborate or complex. Beans, rice, greens (kale and collards), and salsa make a meal, as do vegetable soup and crackers, hummus in a tortilla with 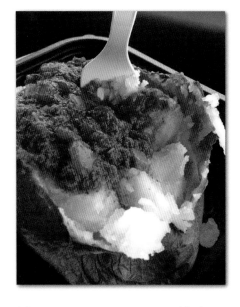 spring mix and tomato, or refried beans with corn, sweet potatoes, and kale. I also love throwing all sorts of things on top of baked potatoes. We make nacho potatoes, "hot dog" potatoes (load up the sauerkraut!), pizza potatoes, and potatoes topped with soup or baked beans.

2 Find a good milk substitute. Every brand is a little different. If you don't like one soy milk, for example, don't assume you won't like *any* brands of soy milk. Try various types and brands as well as sweetened and unsweetened. Soy, almond, and grain milks are the most common nondairy milks. Coconut milk beverages (*not* canned coconut milk) are newer but quickly becoming popular, too. You can also find oat milk, hemp milk, quinoa milk, and a few other varieties at health food stores.

A good place to start is sweetened almond milk, which I find is the most popular option with newbies. If you previously drank skim cow's milk, try rice milk, as it's more diluted than almond or soy milks. Conversely, if you

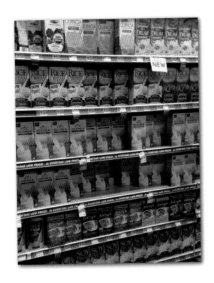

liked whole, full-fat milk, try the coconut milk beverage—it's very thick and creamy. Hemp milk has a bit of a nutty, earthy flavor to it, and oat milk tastes a little like, well, plain oatmeal.

I find soy and almond milks work best for cooking and baking. I generally shy away from coconut because it's high in saturated fat and the taste is strong. (I avoid hemp for that reason, too.) But that's my personal preference. Find a milk—or milks—you can use in all the ways you were using cow's milk to make your plant-based transition a success.

Note that shelf-stable nondairy milks tend to be cheaper than refrigerated nondairy milks (which sometimes contain oil), and you can stock up on them so you never run out. Big bulk retailers like Costco also tend to have bargains. And I once found nondairy milk at the dollar store . . . for $1!

3 Eat starches. Include plenty of whole grains like brown rice and starchy vegetables like potatoes in your diet. These foods will help you feel satisfied and energized. Because vegetables are so low in calories, it's easy to fill up and feel stuffed on few calories, leaving you feeling tired—and hungry soon after. Including grains, potatoes, beans, fruits, and lentils helps prevent this from happening. Additionally, if you're at a healthy weight (or you need to *gain* weight), and you don't have heart disease, type 2 diabetes, or other medical issues, add some high-fat whole plant foods like nuts, seeds, and avocado to your diet.

Whatever you do, don't let yourself go hungry! If you are hungry, eat! Don't worry about portion size. Eat whole plant foods to your heart's content, especially as you transition.

4 Stash snacks everywhere: in your car, purse, laptop bag, locker, desk, and so on. Have plenty of healthy options on hand. (*See "Traveling" in chapter five for ideas.*)

5 Stock up. Stock your fridge and pantry (*see the shopping list in chapter ten, "Getting Started on Your Plant-Based Journey"*), but also buy healthy "convenience" foods for last-minute meals. Purchase canned beans, precooked brown rice, frozen vegetables, pasta, marinara sauce, salsa, tortillas (store in freezer), and refried beans. These nonperishable items can hang out on standby and be on a plate in five minutes when you're starving.

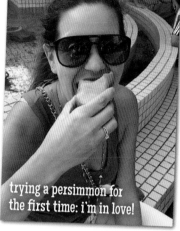

6 Be adventurous. At least once a week try something out of your comfort zone, like a new cuisine or a new ingredient. Make new friends in the produce aisle!

7 Eat freely. Unless you have a medical condition, allow yourself some freedom as you transition. If you want a vegan

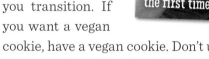

trying a persimmon for the first time: i'm in love!

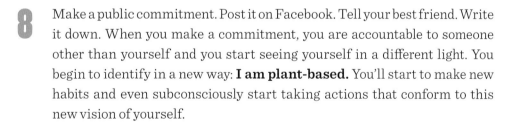

cookie, have a vegan cookie. Don't use your transition period as a free-for-all, but if you can't shake the craving for, say, cheese pizza, make yourself a vegan pizza. (*See "Vegan [Not Plant-Based] Substitutes: Meat, Cheese, Ice Cream, and More" later in this chapter.*)

8 Make a public commitment. Post it on Facebook. Tell your best friend. Write it down. When you make a commitment, you are accountable to someone other than yourself and you start seeing yourself in a different light. You begin to identify in a new way: **I am plant-based.** You'll start to make new habits and even subconsciously start taking actions that conform to this new vision of yourself.

9 Network. Seek out a vegan meet-up group or vegetarian society in your area. Make friends online—join Happy Herbivore's Facebook page or start a blog or a Twitter, Pinterest, or Instagram account. If you don't have Herbie friends locally, you'll have them online! If you want to be my friend, look for @happyherbivore on social media. Many other Herbies also use the hashtag #happyherbivore—it's an easy way to find new friends online.

10 Sign up for the meal plans. My 7-Day Meal Plans (http://www.getmealplans. com) are perfect for newbies—they really take out all the guesswork and they're suitable for all diets, including gluten-free, soy-free, and nut- and seed-free. Try it for a week or make a longer commitment. New, seasonal meal plans are released each week, and they come with recipes and a shopping list. Having a plan makes it so much easier to eat healthy.

common objections

I've already addressed some of the more common myths about a plant-based lifestyle in chapter one, which clears up many of the doubts I often hear. But here are some additional topics and common objections I hear regarding the plant-based lifestyle.

objection: "why not 'everything in moderation'?"

"Moderation" is a vague term. What is "in moderation"? Once a week? Once a month? Once a day? Does the standard apply across the board for everything?

Let's face it, any time we've said "in moderation" to ourselves, our friends, to anyone, it was a *justification*. A justification to eat something we know isn't a healthy choice. It's nothing short of an insincere apology, a Hail Mary to save face and feel less guilty.

We deceive ourselves by believing that everything is okay in moderation. (Funny, you never hear that about arsenic!)

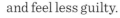

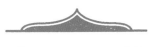

The surest way NOT to fail is to determine to succeed.

—RICHARD SHERIDAN—

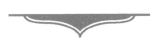

When you make a less-than-great choice, don't *justify* it. Call it what it is: a little indulging. You'll find you indulge less when you think of it this way than you did when operating under the "in moderation" theory. As I'll touch on later with regard to dealing with cravings, here's something that can help: I tell my clients to admit out loud, "I'm not hungry, but I'm going to eat it anyway," or, "I know this doughnut isn't healthy, but I'm going to eat it because I want to."

I strive for 100 percent pure plant perfection, but I have days where I fall to around 85 percent perfect (I'm always vegan, though). I admit that I can't pass up the salty, soft (vegan!) pretzel at a baseball game or Red Vines at the movie theater. Yet I don't tell myself "everything in moderation." I'm indulging and I know it. Plus, there are plenty of foods I don't want to moderate, like vegetables and leafy greens—the more, the better! We all have to find our balance, but strive for the best and when you have a treat, recognize it as a treat.

objection: "can't I just take a supplement?"

I'll refer this one to Dr. Campbell, who says in his book *Whole*: "Recent reductionist research has shown that supplementation doesn't work. As it turns out, an apple does a lot more inside our bodies than all the known apple nutrients ingested in pill form. The whole apple is far more than the sum of its parts."[2]

objection: "eating healthy is expensive!"

Eating plant-based can be deliciously affordable if you stick to the basics—and steer clear of packaged, processed foods. Sure, some premium foods like vegan ice cream are pricey, but the cost is comparable to premium dairy ice cream—and this isn't something you would be buying regularly, anyway.

Even in health food stores you'll find that most of the expensive items are prepared foods (so you're paying for the preparation, just as you pay for the wait service at a nice restaurant) and fancy vegan substitutes, like faux cheese, vegan cookies, or meat analogues. Prepared foods and vegan treats shouldn't be part of your regular grocery bill, or your regular diet, so don't worry about those costs.

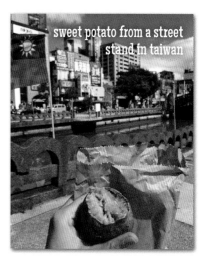

sweet potato from a street stand in taiwan

All healthy, whole plant foods are fairly reasonably priced, especially if you buy in season and/or locally. And don't worry if you can't afford organic—I can't. I like to remind myself that a conventional apple is still healthier than an organic potato chip, and that conventional spinach is better than no spinach at all. **Success with the plant-based diet is more important than ideology.**

Those who adopt a plant-based diet often find they spend *less*, not more, on groceries than they used to. My 7-Day Meal Plan users, for example, spend as little as $30 to $50 per person a week on groceries—for all twenty-one of their meals plus seven snacks and seven desserts.

Nondairy milk (e.g., soy milk, almond milk) is usually cheaper than dairy milk. Beans, lentils, and grains like rice cost a fraction of what you'd pay for even the cheapest slabs of meat. Frozen vegetables are a bargain (my local store sells ten bags for $10!) and you can't beat seasonal fruits on sale.

When my husband and I first adopted a plant-based diet, I cut our grocery bill in half. Nearly every day I have people e-mailing me excitedly about their savings at the grocery store or how they're eating more food but spending less money. I just love loading five and six bags of groceries in my car knowing I didn't spend even $100.

Plus, think about all the money you'll save on health-care costs in the future! Wouldn't you rather spend more money on peas now instead of pills later?

objection: "I want to have my cake and eat it, too."

"You're saying I'll never again be able to [enjoy ice cream on the boardwalk/ grab wings for a game/ participate in family traditions]? These are my 'good times' foods!"

Food is emotional. I get it. Two things to remember: First, you can have a vegan or plant-based version. There is a commercial substitute or recipe for anything you can think of—I promise. Second, you'll make new food memories and new traditions, and your tastes will change. I find the longer you eat a plant-based diet, the less those "foods" appeal to you.

For example, my father was a big meat guy. He loved turkey on Thanksgiving— it was his absolute favorite. Since my mother never cooked turkey the other 364 days a year, he went crazy in November. The first Thanksgiving after he went plant-based (in January, eleven months earlier), I was a little worried how he would fare. He didn't say anything at dinner out of respect for our extended family, but on the car ride home he commented how disgusted he had been looking at the bird on the table and how he had had to excuse himself from the kitchen when my cousins were picking the bird clean—an activity he had enjoyed a year earlier.

Another thought: Do we really want to make life about the food and not the experiences we're having? Isn't it the time with our family and friends that makes eating special? My entire immediate family is plant-based now (it took years of convincing!) and we are making new memories and starting new traditions. And now we'll live longer and better and have more years together, which is what matters most. I wish so much that my grandparents could have seen me grow into the person I am today. I lost them right after high school to Western diseases. My parents and I share a lot of grief, wishing we had known then what we know now.

objection: "I'm a picky eater. I don't like [long list of plant foods]. I hate vegetables."

I was horribly picky when I was an omnivore. I can remember going to a restaurant with my husband and being near tears at the table because nothing appealed to me. Those days are long gone. It's not just me—I hear this story

FIVE STAGES OF GRIEF

All change is grief, and changing long-held patterns can be painful. As you progress through your plant-based journey, you may find yourself experiencing the five stages of grief:

DENIAL: "If this was true, I would have heard about it on the news." "I don't really need to make a drastic change. My grandmother lived to be a hundred and ate like me."

ANGER: "I can't believe how much misinformation is out there. Marketing unhealthy products as healthy should be illegal!"

BARGAINING: "I'll only cheat when I go out to dinner . . . or it's my birthday . . . or . . ."

DEPRESSION: "I'll never again have [insert beloved unhealthy food here]?" "How can I live without cheese?"

ACCEPTANCE: "I love being plant-based! I only wish I'd known about this and done this sooner."

The good news: Everyone makes their way to the acceptance stage eventually. You just have to stick with it!

ROBIN: LOST MORE THAN 200 POUNDS
december 2012

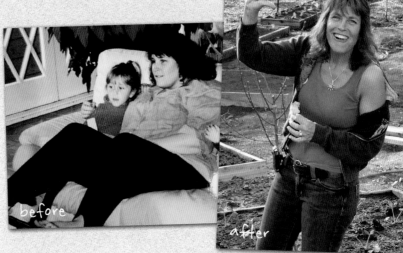
before

after

HH: Two hundred pounds is an incredible weight loss! Tell us about that.

I am more embarrassed about my weight loss than proud of it. I mean, how can a person let themselves get up to 333 pounds? I have tried to hide the fact that I have lost 201 pounds, because telling someone that is like saying I was a failure. I know it is a backward way of thinking, but I have a lot of shame about ever being that big. I think unless you have ever been that overweight, you don't realize how alone and alienated you feel by being the largest person in a room, or not fitting into normal clothes.

HH: So what happened? How did you get up to 333 pounds?

I have always struggled with my weight throughout my life. When I was a child, my mother was a health nut and completely obsessed with her weight (and mine). She convinced me that I was a fat kid and I was always being restricted or put on a diet. The funny thing is, when I look back at old pictures of myself as a child, I had a normal weight and was not heavy at all. I did eventually gain weight when I was in middle school and high school and was sent to fat camps during the summer, where I would lose 30 pounds, get back down to a normal weight, and then gain it back during the school year. I used food as a friend, to comfort me when I felt alone.

I finally found love when I was twenty years old and I dealt with all the ups and downs of that relationship by using food as my drug of choice. Eleven years later, my marriage ended. Since I was thin, I couldn't blame it on my weight, which I had always done in the past. That *sucked*! I always had told myself that if I were just thin, then my life would be perfect. Wrong!!! My weight went up and down most of my adult life, but my divorce sent me over the deep end. Because I wasn't fat when my marriage ended, it must be me that was flawed. At least that was what I told myself at the time. I drowned myself in food. No one was ever going to get that close to me and hurt me again. I went from 135 pounds to 333 pounds. I had given up! At least I thought I had.

HH: What changed?

One day, I went to pick my daughter up at her girlfriend's house. She lived on top of a very steep hill and I had to park my car at the bottom and walk up. By the time I got to the front door, I thought I was having a heart attack. I was beet red, I couldn't stop sweating, and I couldn't catch my breath. I thought, "This is insane!" I am killing myself and I have a four-year-old daughter to take care of. Time to change! They say it matters why we end up fat and that we are eating to stuff down some big emotions that we don't want to deal with. That's probably true, but in the end for me it just all boiled down to the fact that I just didn't want to live like this anymore. I didn't want my daughter to grow up with a mom who she had to make excuses for, and I didn't want her to turn out like me.

HH: What did you do? Did you change your diet? Exercise?

I am somewhat of an extremist (it takes that all-or-nothing personality to get up to 333 pounds), so I decided to pick a diet that was the complete opposite of the way I was eating. I was living on coffee, diet soda, candy, ice cream, and fast food. So, I then chose a diet that eliminated all processed food, all caffeine, and all bread, and the only carbs I ate were fruits and vegetables. I slowly started exercising again. At first I could only do five minutes on a stationary bike, but that was a start. I worked my way up to forty-five minutes. If I wanted to overeat, I turned to chicken, cheese, and salad with olive oil and balsamic vinegar. Even with the overeating, I still lost weight. In about two years, I was down to 165 pounds, but the scale stopped moving.

HH: What brought you to a plant-based diet?

After the weight loss I felt really good, but I still had 30 pounds left to go, and I knew the large amounts of chicken and cheese I was eating weren't that healthy. For the first time in my life, I stopped focusing on the weight and started focusing on my health. I read a book that advocated a vegan diet but was afraid that the main reason the cravings were gone was because all that protein was stabilizing my blood sugar. Still, I felt it was something I had to try, so I eliminated all animal products and added more carbs in the form of beans and whole grains like quinoa, yams, sweet potatoes, corn, and rice.

HH: What was the result?

I was right, the cravings came back, but I fought through them and managed to lose 20 more pounds. I was down to 145 pounds, but I was fighting back the urge to overeat all the time.

HH: Did it ever get better for you?

After a couple of years of being vegan, I lost all desire to eat animal products. My big problem was that slowly but surely, my desire for sugar was creeping its way back. Sugar is vegan, you know. Over the next few years, I managed to keep almost all of the weight off with the exception of 25 pounds that I would keep losing by juice fasting, or worse, the Master Cleanse (a concoction of lemon juice, cayenne pepper, and maple syrup), and regaining by bingeing on sugar and fat. I would rationalize my action by telling myself at least when I was overeating, I was eating the healthy version of unhealthy foods like organic chocolate instead of a Hershey bar, or healthy cookies with agave nectar and oil instead of an Oreo, or raw chocolate treats with nuts and coconut oil. I was losing my war on controlling my cravings and I was scared to death of gaining my weight back. I had made a promise to myself that I would never let that happen, but I seemed to think 20 to 30 pounds still kept me within a normal weight range, so it was okay.

HH: Was there another turning point for you?

The next turning point for me came during a family trip to Disneyland. We were in Tomorrowland and they had an exhibit showing what 10 pounds of human fat looks like, and it hit me. I was carrying around two to three extra of those unhealthy, jelly-looking things with me.

I decided the juice fasting was becoming more unhealthy than healthy for me, because I was using it as an easy way to lose weight fast, and then I would go back to bingeing on sugar and unhealthy (yet vegan), processed, fat-laden foods soon afterward. I was fed up and ready to get off this ride. So this time, I tried green smoothies. I thought for me they were healthier because they had the fiber, but they were also high in fat (nuts) and sugar (dates and fruit). It wasn't until I watched the movie *Forks Over Knives* and saw Dr. Esselstyn speak that a bell went off and I *finally* got it. It was the fat that was

continued on page 130

TIPS FOR PLANT-BASED EATING ON A BUDGET

» **Stick to basics.** You can create varied and healthy meals with simple basics like grains, beans, lentils, seasonal fruits, and vegetables.

» **Buy in bulk.** Use the bulk bins at your store, buy in bulk online (try Bulkfoods.com, Vitacost.com, or Amazon.com), look for deals at bulk stores (like Costco), and buy the biggest option (i.e., 5-pound bag of rice instead of a 1-pound bag). Buy a bag of potatoes or a bag of onions instead of one or two at a time. Remember: You pay a premium for anything premeasured or scaled down to a single portion. For example, you can get a huge tub of oats that'll last months for the same price as six packets of instant oatmeal in a box.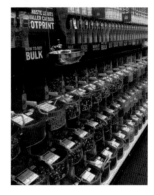

» **Get ethnic.** Shop at ethnic markets in your area. I find amazing deals at the Asian supermarket and Indian grocery store in my town. I can buy a bag of lentils the size of a pillowcase for $5! The ethnic aisle at the supermarket has great deals, too. For example, spices, rice, and beans are much cheaper on the ethnic aisle than on the other aisles!

» **Buy generic.**

» **Shop around.** It's not the most convenient, but it's a great way to save money. Find out which stores have the best prices and keep up on sales. Sometimes non-grocery retail stores like Target or Walmart have the best prices on food, especially if you're willing to buy a bigger quantity or size.

» **Distinguish between staple and convenience food.** I always thought canned beans were a staple when really they're just more convenient. I can buy a bag of dry beans that will last for several meals for the price of one can of beans. (Cook a big batch of beans and rice and freeze in 1-cup portions for later.)

» **Try the health food store.** Health food stores get a reputation for being expensive, and some of their premium and prepared foods can be (again, convenience fees), but there are plenty of bargains, too. Spices, for example, tend to be much cheaper at my Whole Foods Market than any of the supermarkets in the area. I also find that, at supermarkets, foods considered to be health foods, like soy milk, are more expensive than at the health food store. Health food stores tend to have more variety, too, and often have huge bulk-bin sections, unlike most supermarkets.

» **Stick to a meal plan.** Create your own or use my 7-Day Meal Plans (http://www.getmealplans.com). Having a plan ensures you only buy what you need. You can also pick recipes that are similar to one another, so you have no spoils or leftovers.

» **Save veggie scraps to make broth.** Watch my how-to broth-making video on HappyHerbivore.com. Freeze one-cup portions as well as "ice cubes" of broth for cooking.

» **Keep it simple with kitchen tools.** You don't need an avocado peeler or a $400 blender to be healthy. All you need are some basics: pots, pans, measuring cups and spoons, a good knife, spatula, whisk, cutting board, mixing bowl, and a cheap blender or food processor. (That's all I had when I wrote *Everyday Happy Herbivore* while living in St. Maarten. You don't need much!) I like to remind myself that some of the healthiest populations barely have electricity. If you want to splurge on specialty tools, do it—but don't feel obligated.

time and time again. Once you start eating real foods, your body wakes up. You'll fall in love with new foods and rediscover old foods you didn't think you liked!

objection: "but I can't live without [product]!"

If I said I couldn't live without heroin, what would you advise? Don't let food control you. Break the addiction. Fight the seduction. Isn't your health—your life—worth it?

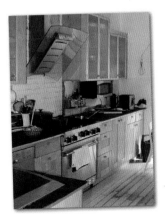

objection: "cooking takes too much time."

I can make a bean burrito in less than thirty seconds— time me! There are so many plant-based options that are faster than fast food (which isn't even all that fast when you add up the time it takes to drive there, wait in line, get the food, and drive home). You can make a PB&J faster than it takes to walk to your car parked in the driveway.

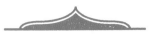

The grand essentials of happiness are: something to do, something to love, and something to hope for.

—ALAN CHALMERS—

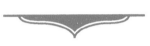

Frozen vegetables and precooked grains—these are all super fast. Then you have beans—they're as fast as it takes you to use a can opener. Don't over-think it. Besides, even if some things take a little longer to make, isn't your health—your life—worth an extra five minutes?

When you do cook, cook more than you need right away, so you have leftovers. Soups are awesome like that.

objection: "we all have to die of something, right?"

Yes, we do, but there are better ways to go. I have watched loved ones waste away from cancer and suffer through terminal illness. I love myself too much to put myself through that, or put my family or friends through it. Watching someone you love suffer when you can't do anything for them is the worst feeling. Plus there is something to be said for *quality* of life. And once you know what it feels like to be well and thrive, you'll do anything to prevent feeling sick again!

objection: "I don't have willpower."

Yes, you do. Dig deep. Find your reasons. Believe them. Prove yourself wrong. You're not weak—you're strong. You *can* do this. Remember, attitude is everything.

Don't be the person telling yourself you can't do something, because as long as you keep saying it, it's going to be true.

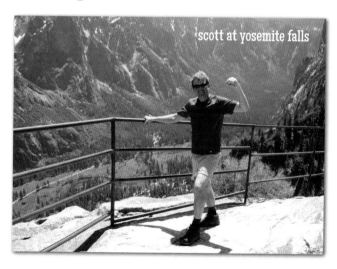

scott at yosemite falls

SALLY: LATE-STAGE OVARIAN CANCER SURVIVOR
november 2013

HH: What made you adopt a plant-based diet?

My "wake-up call" came shockingly and abruptly—in August 2007, I was diagnosed with late-stage ovarian cancer. I was especially stunned because I considered myself to be in excellent health; that is, I ate a low-fat diet (which, of course, included lots of dairy products, eggs, and poultry), exercised regularly, maintained a healthy weight, and followed through with recommended health-care checkups and screenings.

HH: What happened after your diagnosis?

Immediately I had surgery, followed by chemotherapy, which put me into remission. However, I was ever-vigilant about if and when the cancer would return. Ovarian cancer is notorious for being diagnosed at an advanced stage, because of the subtlety of symptoms and lack of reliable screening tests, and stubbornly recurring after remission.

HH: What led you to a plant-based diet?

In 2008, I read an interview with David Servan-Schreiber, a busy doctor and neuroscientist who found out that he had a brain tumor at age thirty-one. In his book, *Anticancer: A New Way of Life*, he detailed the roles that nutrition, along with environmental toxins, physical activity, and emotional health, have in keeping cancer at bay. This book opened my eyes to the relationship between foods and health; as Servan-Schreiber stated: "Every day at every meal we can choose the food that will defend our bodies against the invasion of cancer." Finally, I had a tool (i.e., food) that could help me fend off cancer resurgence—what an empowering feeling! Realizing that the foods consumed on a day-to-day basis have an immediate and lasting impact on health and well-being, I began my journey into the realm of plant-based eating. I have never looked back.

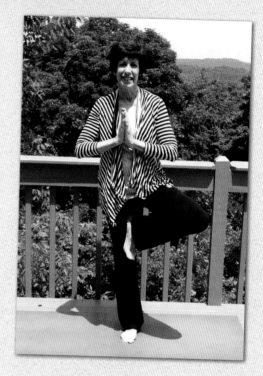

HH: What's your diet like now?

For my daily eating regimen, I refer to Dr. Campbell's guidelines for daily calories: 80 percent from complex carbohydrates, 10 percent from protein, and 10 percent from fat. Eating whole plant foods definitely has changed my taste buds—I never thought that I would be craving fresh arugula in my morning oatmeal! Although I still have my daily piece of 72 percent dark chocolate, I cringe at the sweetness of most desserts and processed foods; I'll eat a baked yam over a piece of cake any day! Plus, the description of sugar as "the fuel of cancer cells" keeps my sweet tooth in check.

In no way do I miss animal foods, especially the dairy products that I used to consume daily. I view food differently now. I consider food to be tasteful, delicious, nourishing, multicolored medicine for my body.

continued on page 130

commercial substitutes

The following lists include brands I recommend as well as vegan substitutes that aren't as healthy.

Ultimately, my advice is to focus your diet around whole, unprocessed plant foods, and to keep the more processed and less healthy vegan alternatives to a minimum. If you decide to incorporate vegan commercial substitutes, let them accent your healthy diet, not be a key player. Remember, just because it's vegan doesn't mean it's healthy.

Please check the ingredients on any package to confirm the item is vegan, as some brands do have non-vegan items and products are subject to change.

plant-based commercial substitutes (happy herbivore–approved brands)

I'm always getting e-mails asking what brands I use—what brands are plant-based, oil-free, whole-wheat (or gluten-free), and vegan.

Regrettably, brands tend to vary by region, and even within the same city or town, the two or three local chain supermarkets might not carry the same brands or items.

The truth is you have to scan labels and check them scrupulously, but eventually you will know what brands at your store are "safe" (or "clean" as my husband and I like to say) and you'll always look for those first.

I don't personally use every item on this list, but I wanted to compile a list of oil-free, plant-based brands that was as comprehensive as possible.

BROTHS
Kitchen Basics Unsalted Vegetable
   Cooking Stock
Pacific Organic Vegetable Broth

BREADS
Alvarado (some contain oil, most do not)
Dave's Killer Bread (contains seeds)

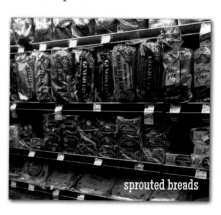

sprouted breads

Ezekiel

Food for Life

TORTILLA/WRAPS

Engine 2 (contains seeds)

Ezekiel

Food for Life

La Tortilla Factory 100-calorie
tortillas

Mission corn tortillas

Sandwichpetals gluten-free tortillas

CRACKERS

Doctor Kracker (contains seeds; not
all varieties are vegan)

Edward & Sons crackers

Engine 2 (contains seeds)

IKEA Crispbreads
(Rye & Multigrain)

La Reina baked unsalted
corn chips

Lundberg brown rice cakes
(some varieties are not vegan)

Manischewitz whole-wheat matzos

Mary's Gone Crackers (contains
nuts or seeds)

Ryvita crackers (some "flavors"
contain oil)

Streit's whole-wheat matzos

Wasa Crackers

Yehuda Matzos

CANNED GOODS

Eden Organics

Muir Glen

Pomi Tomatoes

Westbrae

SPECIALIZED CONDIMENTS

Braggs dressings

Bragg Liquid Aminos

Delallo marinara sauce

Muir Glen organic pasta sauce

DRINKS

Almond Breeze

Silk (some varieties contain oil)

WestSoy

HUMMUS

Cedars Fat-Free (plain and
roasted red pepper)

Engine 2 (contains seeds)

Oasis Naturals Mediterranean
Cuisine

Roots Oil-Free Original

SNACKS

Bearitos Organic No Salt No Oil
microwave popcorn

Food for Lovers Vegan Queso

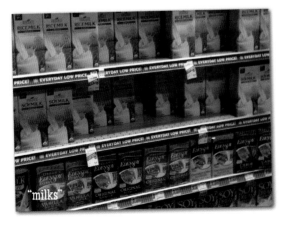
"milks"

Larabars (contains nuts and seeds)

Suncakes

That's It fruit bars

PREPARED FOODS

Eden Organics

McDougall's Right Foods

STORE BRANDS

Trader Joe's

Whole Foods Market

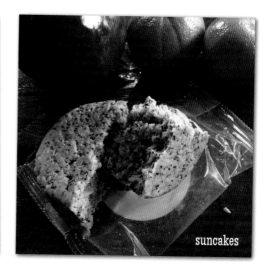
suncakes

vegan (not plant-based) substitutes: meat, cheese, ice cream, and more

My advice to my clients is to not eat vegan analogues right away because (1) they don't taste *the same* and (2) most are not healthful choices and I want my clients to start adjusting to a less processed, more whole foods diet from the start. I want them to stop looking for meat and cheese on their plate. I want them to fall in love with the color, textures, and variety of plant foods. I want them to fill their plates with vegetables, grains, beans, and fruits—not Boca burgers and vegan hot dogs.

However, I have found that some individuals find comfort in knowing they can have an "alternative" and for those people, vegan substitutes can be a comfort during transition. My husband is a great example. He was a cheese fanatic. Life

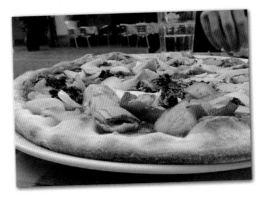

without pizza was no life at all, or so he told me. That's when I made him a vegan cheese pizza, and once he had it, he realized going completely dairy-free was possible. He could have his cake—er, pizza—and eat it, too. As time went on, my husband ate less and less of the vegan cheese and now he rarely eats it at all.

Similarly, a friend found it much easier to transition her kids to a plant-based diet if they were still allowed vegan chicken nuggets once a week as a treat. "You've got to pick your battles!" she told me, and I couldn't agree more.

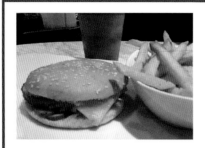

A diet of vegan burgers and fries, vegan chicken tenders, and potato chips is only marginally better than the drive-thru. That's not optimum. I want my clients to thrive. I want them to overhaul their diet to regain their health, not just "veganize" it.

It's all about progress, not perfection. I respect that not everyone can do a total 180 from the Standard American Diet to pure plant perfection (I couldn't). Some of us need baby steps and that's okay. Do the best you can. If the training wheels keep you from failing and quitting and help you get to where you ultimately want to go, that's okay with me.

My diet is much healthier today than it was even a year ago. I keep making better changes and choices with time. The journey never ends!

PETA (People for the Ethical Treatment of Animals) maintains an Accidentally Vegan Food List you can check out (it was much too long to reprint here). It includes Ritz crackers, Club crackers, and Oreos, just to name a few.

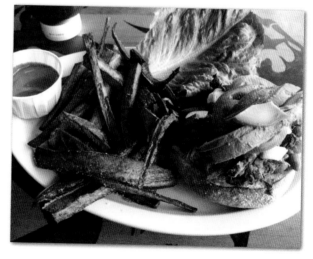

Note that I have traveled quite a bit throughout Europe and, where possible, I've included brands of vegan products I found abroad.

NONDAIRY MILKS AND CREAMERS

Almond Breeze

Alpro Soya (EU)

Rice Dream

Silk

So Delicious

WestSoy

YOGURT AND PUDDING

Almond Dream

Alpro Soya (EU)

Amande

Danone Savia (EU)

Provamel (EU)

Ricera

Silk

Sojade (EU)

Sojasun (EU)

Trader Joe's

WayFare

WholeSoy & Co.

Wildwood

ZenSoy

CHEESE AND SOUR CREAM

Cheezly by Redwood

Daiya

Dr-Cow's Tree Nut Cheese

Follow Your Heart

Food for Lovers Vegan Queso

Galaxy Nutritional Foods/
   GO Veggie!

Nacheez

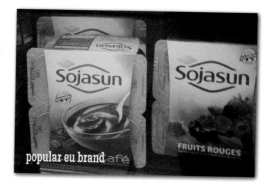

popular eu brand

Nacho Mom's Cheese Sauce

Parma!

Road's End Organics Cheese

Road's End Organics Nacho
   Cheese Dip

Sheese (UK)

Sunergia Soyfoods Soy Feta

Teese

Tofutti

Trader Joe's (cream cheese
   and shreds)

WayFare We Can't Say It's Cheese

MEAT SUBSTITUTES

365 (Whole Foods Market)

Amy's

Asherah's Gourmet (oil-free,
   contains coconut and seeds)

Beyond Meat

Boca

Cactus Jerky (oil-free)

Cluckphrey

Field Roast

Gardein

Gardenburger
Gimme Lean (oil-free)
Lightlife (Smart) (some
    oil-free)
Match Meats
Moophrey
MorningStar Farms
Nate's Meatballs
Primal Strips (some oil-free)
Quorn
Sophie's Kitchen
Sunshine Burger (oil-free, may
    contain nuts or seeds)
Tofu Pups
Tofurkey
Trader Joe's
Upton's Naturals (oil-free)
Vegetarian Plus
VegeUSA
WestSoy seitan
Yves (some oil-free)

CONDIMENTS AND DRESSINGS
Amy's
El Paso Enchilada Sauce
Follow Your Heart
Hershey's Syrup
Nasoya
Spectrum
Trader Joe's Reduced Fat
    Mayonnaise
Vegenaise

FROZEN DINNERS AND PIZZAS
Amy's
Candle Cafe
Dr. Praeger's (some contain eggs)
Health Is Wealth
Ian's
Kashi
Tofurkey
Tofutti
Trader Joe's
Vegetarian Plus

FROZEN WAFFLES
Nature's Path
Trader Joe's
Vans

ICE CREAM
Luna & Larry's
Purely Decadent
Rice Dream
So Delicious
Soy Dream

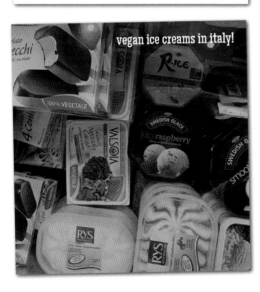

vegan ice creams in italy!

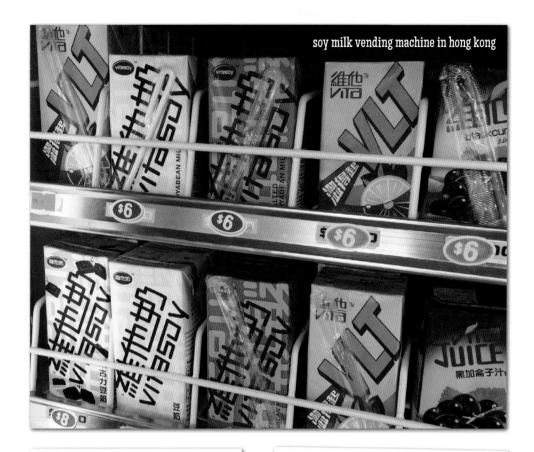
soy milk vending machine in hong kong

Temptation
Tofutti

SNACK BARS AND MEAL BARS
BumbleBar
Clif Bar
Enjoy Life
Gnu Foods
Kind
Lärabar
Luna
Odwalla
Oskri

ProBar
Pure Bar
Organic Food Bar
Raw Revolution
Keen-Wäh (oil-free)

CANDY—MADE SPECIALLY VEGAN
Annie's Fruit Snacks
Dandies
Lenny & Larry's
Go Max Go
Surf Sweets
Sweet & Sara

minimalist meals

Just because I write cookbooks for a living doesn't mean I always love to cook. I love simple meals—a lot. I have days where I can't be bothered to cook. I just want to heat something up and be done with it. I'm slightly embarrassed to admit how often those days happen!

Living in St. Maarten, where "eating out" and precooked vegan food was off the menu, I got into the habit of making simpler meals. That's what *Everyday Happy Herbivore*, the book I wrote while I lived there, is all about, but here is a formula that's even simpler:

grain/potato + bean/tofu + greens/veg + sauce

Yep. It's that easy.

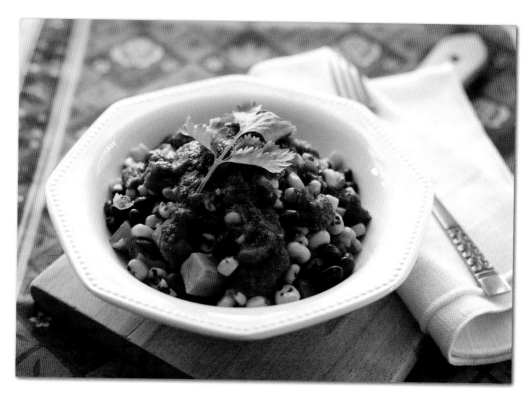

Here are some examples of taking this simple formula (or slight variations of it) to make a meal:

brown rice + black beans + kale + pineapple or peach salsa

quinoa + white beans + baby spinach + strawberries + balsamic dressing

pasta + chickpeas + broccoli + marinara sauce

tortilla + spinach + tomato + hummus

quinoa + chickpeas + bell pepper + italian dressing

sweet potato + black beans + corn + enchilada sauce

potato + chickpeas + kale + gravy

brown rice + black-eyed peas + corn + bbq sauce

brown rice + tofu or edamame + frozen mixed vegetables + soy sauce

quinoa + tempeh + pineapple + teriyaki sauce

You can expand on any of these by adding sliced green onions or diced red onion, or another vegetable (cherry tomatoes pretty much go with anything)—or, if you're not eating a low-fat diet, nuts, seeds, and avocado.

If you can open a can, you can make these meals—and you can make them in the time it takes you to open the can. You can find precooked grains (like quinoa or brown rice) on the shelf or freezer of any store, and they take a minute or two to heat up. Canned beans just need a rinse. The vegetables might need a moment in the microwave or steamer and the same for the sauces.

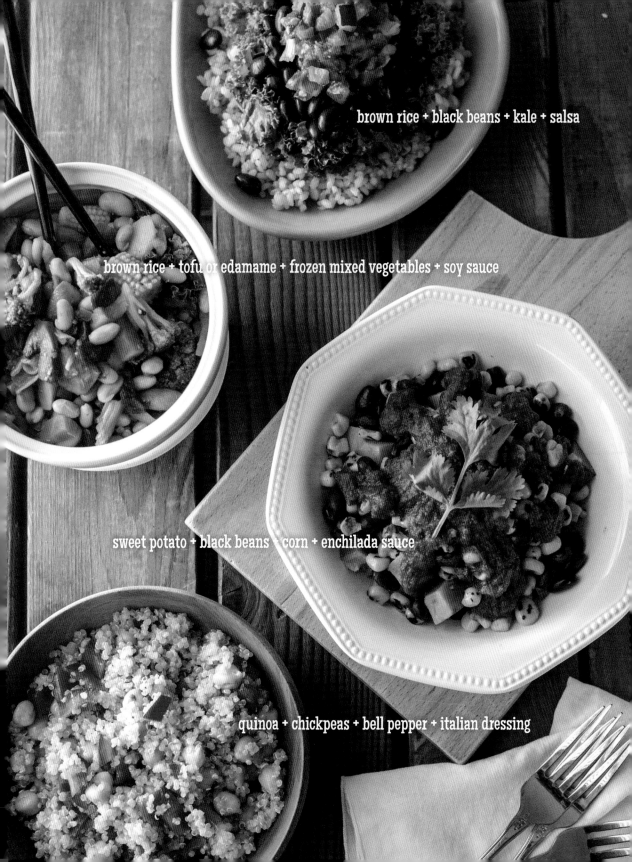

brown rice + black beans + kale + salsa

brown rice + tofu or edamame + frozen mixed vegetables + soy sauce

sweet potato + black beans + corn + enchilada sauce

quinoa + chickpeas + bell pepper + italian dressing

Robin's story continued from page 115

addictive! I thought it was the sugar and the carbs, but fruit alone or grains without fat are *not* addictive.

HH: What's your diet like now?

Now I follow a no-oil, no-nuts, fat-free, plant-based diet with *lots* of greens, and I'm the thinnest (132 pounds) I have ever been. I love the way I feel and how weight (and food obsession) is no longer a problem for me.

I am also really happy that I persuaded my husband and daughter to eat this way as well. My husband has suffered from knee problems for the past fifteen years and hasn't been able to run or ride bicycles for the last ten. He assumed it was from years of abuse from being a carpet layer and a previous motorcycle accident. After a month of eating this way, he ran up the driveway and got all the way to the house before he noticed he was running (no pain),

and we just went on a seventeen-mile bike ride a few weeks ago. Before switching to this way of eating, he was looking into knee replacement surgery.

HH: When I first saw your pictures, I could not believe you are fifty. Fifty is a big birthday for a lot of people—was it for you?

When I turned fifty, I did some real soul-searching. It was a hard birthday, because I felt I was saying good-bye to the last fifty years, and then I realized that wasn't true. I was actually saying "HELLO" to the next fifty. I had been designing T-shirts and products for everyone else over the last twenty-five years and decided to follow my passion. So I came up with a line of vegan tees and gifts. I am so passionate about this lifestyle and way of eating, and I feel it has changed every aspect of my life. I am vegan for life!

Sally's story continued from page 119

HH: Do you believe being plant-based has helped keep the cancer at bay?

Fewer than 50 percent of the women with advanced-stage ovarian cancer live five years after diagnosis. I am one of the fortunate survivors—six years after diagnosis, I remain cancer-free. I am convinced that adopting a plant-based diet, along with a routine that includes yoga, family, friends, and loads of gratitude, keeps me cancer-free.

The more I read about and experience whole food, plant-based nutrition, the more passionate I have become about advocating this lifestyle to others. I strive to inform and support fellow ovarian cancer survivors about how they can use food as a powerful weapon in their journey toward healing and long-term health.

I became a plant-based advocate after diagnosis of late-stage ovarian cancer six years ago. I am convinced about the powerful effects of eating whole plant-based foods to heal from and protect against cancer. My passion now is to spread the word to other ovarian cancer survivors, and you have helped me do just that!

UPDATE (summer 2014):

Seven years after diagnosis, I remain cancer-free. Also, I am expanding my educational outreach to others by leading presentations, workshops, and a local support group for plant-based eating. Each day, I put into practice the message of Food for Health (a nonprofit that I created): eating as if your life depends on it!

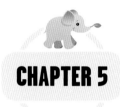

plant-based life on-the-go

"If you do what you need, you're surviving. If you do what you want, you're living."

—UNKNOWN—

I find the biggest worry newcomers have is how their diet will work socially. (*See "Social Situations" in chapter six for more on this.*) The second biggest concern is how it will work outside the home, especially while traveling.

I recently walked into a roadhouse in Wyoming. The special of the day was bone marrow (I'm really not joking). I was sure this place might finally beat me, but I was delighted to find an Ebony & Ivory salad on the menu that was not only plant-based, but also oil-free. I nearly died. (And it was so delicious that I went back the very next day!) Some of the best vegan meals I've had have been in roadhouses and steak houses! Don't judge a book by its cover and a restaurant by its... *erm,* decor.

eating out

I've traveled all over the United States—including to tiny towns in remote areas—as well as internationally, and I've never had trouble foraging for plant-based fare. Sure, I've had to get a little creative at times (and occasionally my meal was pretty boring), but I've always found something to eat and I've had some pretty remarkable experiences (and meals!) along the way.

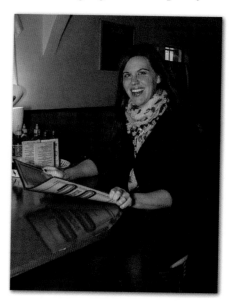

But before we get to the part where I tell you how to find something to eat, we have to get something out of the way first:

You are not a burden.

Don't be shy in asking for what you want (or explaining what you don't want). Remember: You're paying a premium to have a meal made your way to order. The restaurant wants your money. It's okay to let them earn it.

Overall, I find most restaurants and wait staff are more than happy to help you. With all the different dietary restrictions and known food allergies today, most chefs and wait staff are used to special requests and having to tweak things. Be polite, smile, say "Thank you" at least twice, and leave a good tip. If I can, I also take five minutes to talk to the manager to tell him or her how happy and satisfied I was with my dining experience.

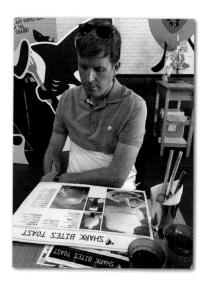

Bonus points: I've had managers take $20 off my bill, thanking me for my feedback. I've had chefs come to my table, saying how much they enjoyed the opportunity to be creative and try something new. One restaurant even put the meal I "created" on their menu! So don't feel like you're a burden—you're not! Plus, your health is more important than the opinion of someone you'll probably never see again, right? Right!

finding options

First, scan the menu to see what you can eat. Is there a vegetarian option that would be vegan if you just left off the cheese or egg? Is there a vegetable-heavy dish that would be plant-based if you just left off the meat? Ask yourself, "*What can be adapted?*"

You can also make your own dish by pulling various other menu items together. Take a look at the side dishes. Can they be made into a meal? Do other dishes have components you might like?

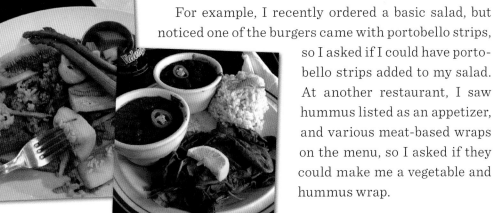

For example, I recently ordered a basic salad, but noticed one of the burgers came with portobello strips, so I asked if I could have portobello strips added to my salad. At another restaurant, I saw hummus listed as an appetizer, and various meat-based wraps on the menu, so I asked if they could make me a vegetable and hummus wrap.

It might take a little creativity on your part, but you'll find some really awesome meals this way. If you're stumped or too intimidated, ask the wait staff and kitchen for help.

veg-friendly cuisines

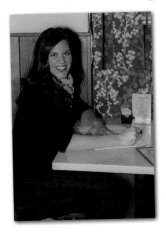

The following types of restaurants tend to have vegetarian sections (or vegetarian items) on their menus. Since these restaurants usually also serve meat, they can be a great middle-ground option when you're the only plant eater in the group. Nevertheless, there are a few things you need to look out for, or keep in mind when ordering, to ensure your meal is vegan, so I've included "what to order" and "what to avoid" for each type of restaurant mentioned here. Also note that many fast-food and chain restaurants are veg-friendly. (*See "Traveling" later in this chapter for details on fast-food establishments you can walk into confidently.*)

MEXICAN

what to order: Burritos, enchiladas, rice and beans, chips and salsa, guacamole, vegetable fajitas. Many places will also substitute beans for meat in any meat dish at no extra charge.

what to avoid: Non-vegetarian beans and rice. Beans could be cooked in lard or animal fat, and rice may be cooked with chicken or beef broth; ask if the rice and beans are vegetarian.

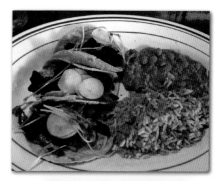

ASIAN

what to order: Vegetable dishes like stir-fries or curries, vegetable sushi, fresh vegetable spring or summer rolls, steamed vegetable dumplings. If you see a meat dish that sounds interesting, ask if they could make it for you with tofu or more vegetables, instead of the meat.

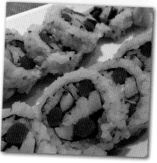

what to avoid: Fish sauce, a common item. When ordering, say "No fish sauce."

INDIAN

what to order: Vegetable or lentil dishes. Most Indian restaurants have a huge vegetarian section on the menu, since many people in India are vegetarian.

what to avoid: Clarified butter (ghee), cream, or cheese. Make sure what you're ordering doesn't contain these dairy items.

ITALIAN

what to order: Pasta, salads, vegetable dishes.

what to avoid: Non-vegan pasta. Inquire whether the pasta contains milk or eggs. (Unless it's fresh pasta, it shouldn't.)

PIZZERIAS

what to order: Cheese-less vegetable pizza.

what to avoid: Crusts or sauce with milk. Most pizzerias do not use milk or dairy in their crust or marinara, but some, like Pizza Hut, do. Inquire before ordering. If the pizza isn't safe, make a jumbo salad from all the toppings.

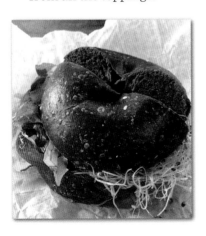

BAGEL AND SANDWICH SHOPS

what to order: A sandwich with every vegetable they have and mustard (or hummus if available). One of my favorite on-the-go meals is a whole-wheat bagel with lettuce, tomato, onion, and yellow mustard. Every bagel shop on the planet has that!

what to avoid: Non-vegan bread. Bread and bagels are usually vegan, but it never hurts to ask.

GRILLS/AMERICAN

what to order: Pepper fajitas, nachos without cheese or sour cream and extra vegetables, grilled vegetables. If they have vegetarian chili, order it without cheese and sour cream and have it dumped over a baked potato or nacho chips. Most restaurant veggie burgers are not vegan, but some are, so do ask.

what to avoid: Toppings with dairy. Make sure to specify, "Hold the cheese and sour cream."

finding healthy options—anywhere

I confess, it's much easier to find something that is vegan than oil-free/plant-based, and eating out (and traveling) may be one of those times that you allow a little vegan junk food or oil back into your otherwise healthy diet. (I admit to having a vegan doughnut on vacation in Portland and vegan gelato in Italy on my birthday.) Nevertheless, if you want to eat as healthy as possible all the time, you can.

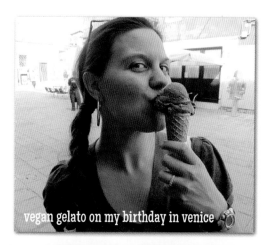
vegan gelato on my birthday in venice

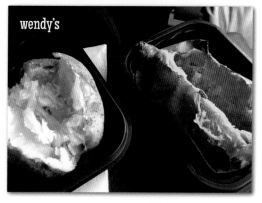
wendy's

At any type of restaurant—even a veg-unfriendly one—you can usually opt for salad, baked potato, and/or steamed vegetables like broccoli. Say it with me: "I can find a salad and a plain baked potato anywhere—even at Wendy's." Though let's hope it doesn't always come to that!

TIPS FOR FINDING HEALTHY OPTIONS ON ANY MENU

» Study the menu for dishes that sound like they could be low-fat (oil-free) and healthy, which means skipping past anything that's fried. I look for items that can be steamed or are not cooked—fresh rolls at a Thai restaurant, for example.

» Inquire whether your meal can be made without oil. Stir-fry dishes can usually be steamed instead of cooked in oil. (At Denny's, for example, you can usually order the stir-fry "dry"—which means cooked without oil.) Grilled vegetable dishes can also generally be prepared without oil if you ask.

» Dress it up. Instead of dressings, try using lemon juice (ask for fresh lemons), hot sauce, or balsamic vinegar. I often carry a tiny spray bottle of Bragg Liquid Aminos with me (it's a little like soy sauce), which is amazing with fresh lemon on a salad. Fresh orange or lime slices are another option, and salsa works great, too! A friend of mine combines Dijon mustard with honey for a honey-mustard dressing. (Most restaurants have honey and mustard.)

» Opt for a salad when in doubt. Salads are always a safe bet when eating out, and if the salad normally comes with meat, ask if you can substitute avocado instead. (California Pizza Kitchen does this at no extra charge.)

» Scavenge at buffets! Recently I was dragged to a "Chinese buffet," which consisted of rows and rows of battered, fried food. They didn't even have a salad bar. Eventually I located rice, green onions, soy sauce, pickled ginger, and pineapple chunks at the dessert bar. I made myself pineapple rice and it was actually pretty delicious! Halfway through, someone brought me Asian hot sauce and it took my meal to another tasty level.

» Look to the sides. Healthy options also tend to lurk in the side dishes: side house salad, steamed vegetables, rice, beans, or a plain baked potato. Order them all.

» Do the best you can in the circumstances you're in—don't pine for utopia. You're not always going to have the best of the best or the most optimal options. Do what you can. Remember: A plate of steamed vegetables and white rice, while not as healthful as brown rice, is still better than a deep-fried spring roll.

AARON: PLANT-BASED FIREFIGHTER
(may 2012)

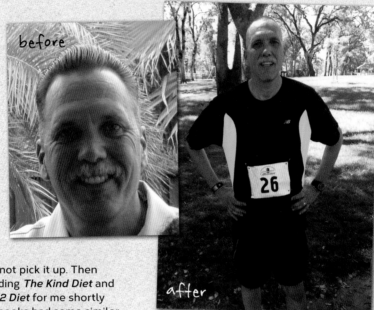

before

after

HH: Since you're a firefighter, I have to ask: Was *The Engine 2 Diet* **instrumental in your transition to a plant-based diet?**

Hearing the information come from a firefighter was probably what drew me to it. I had seen the *Engine 2 Diet* book on a couple of trips to Whole Foods Market and flipped through it, but I did not pick it up. Then my wife started reading *The Kind Diet* and bought *The Engine 2 Diet* for me shortly after that. The two books had some similar thoughts on whole food, plant-based dieting, and that confirmation also helped me decide.

HH: What was your health like before switching to a plant-based diet?

I would call my overall health okay. I was diagnosed with high blood pressure a couple of years ago but had no other major health problems. I took blood pressure meds and was also a little overweight; it was mostly the annoying middle-aged male belly fat. The big push came when I was put on statin drugs for high cholesterol after my last physical.

HH: You recently had your first physical since going plant-based, right? How'd that go?

I just had a physical two weeks ago, and I was expecting to get a scolding from my doctor since I took myself off the statins, but my cholesterol numbers were even better than when I was on the statin drugs!

He also took me off my blood-pressure meds, and I've lost 22 pounds as well.

HH: I was really moved by the camaraderie among the firefighters of Engine 2. Do you find a lot of support from other firefighters?

My crew has been patient with me. It is a team effort. If they cook something with meat, they will either serve the meat on the side, or I will just eat the side dishes. Usually, the side dishes are a salad, pasta, or a rice dish. Dairy dishes are more of a challenge, but when we had enchiladas recently, I made some with vegan cheese. Occasionally I will have some of what they serve. I did have a small piece of steak for a crew member's birthday dinner. *Shhh. It was small. Don't tell Rip!* My crew does give me a little lighthearted grief. If I have trouble with a task, they tell me it is because I have given up meat.

HH: Have you cooked some plant-based meals for your crew? How did that go?

I have made a couple. I have been told that if I cook and eat it, then they will eat it. I just need to build up my arsenal of recipes. I may also make meat on the side for them when I cook. As you can see from some of these answers, meat is a staple in a lot of firehouse meals. In fact, most shopping trips start in the meat section. They get the meat they are going to have that night and then build out from there.

HH: The biggest piece of advice I offer is "plan ahead." Bring plenty of food with you. However, your schedule can be very unpredictable and you probably can't carry a snack bag either. Is it hard for you to stay plant-based while working?

There are days when we run all day and I have not had a chance to shop or cook a meal. Those become pizza nights. They are few and far between. Last time we had a pizza night, I was able to find enough food to get by without partaking in the pizza. That was tough. I love pizza. Sometimes necessity requires that I eat what is available. When that happens, I try to stick as close to vegan as possible, but in this business that can be difficult. I tell people I am 90 to 95 percent vegan.

Another challenge comes when I work at another station on another shift. I usually take extra food and will eat that if they are having a meal that involves meat, dairy, and/or eggs. So far, so good.

HH: Any additional comments?

Going from being known as an "Ambassador of Bacon" to a whole food, plant-based (vegan) diet was not easy. If you are considering making the switch to a whole food, plant-based diet, do it slowly. I rushed into it a little quicker than I should have; that wasn't smart. My wife and I did go through and get rid of a lot of junk and processed foods. I still have a weakness for potato chips. I'm working on that.

I also wanted to share that I ran my first marathon in April 2012.

UPDATE (summer 2014):

It has been just over two and half years since going plant-based. I am still 90 to 95 percent vegan, as work and traveling may require otherwise. At home I am 100 percent. I have moved to a new station, and we are making more plant-based meals. Many nights we have no meat or dairy on the table at all. However, my crew recently sent me a picture of their steak dinner while I was on vacation; firehouse humor is great.

My health continues to get better. I recently had a physical, and the physician's assistant I saw said, "Come back when you have something wrong with you."

Since my interview in May 2012, I have participated in the Tough Mudder twice, ran a couple half-marathons, a half-Ironman, and the California International Marathon. I am much more active than I was before changing my lifestyle. I am also talking with many friends and family members about the changes going plant-based have made in my life. It is great to see some of them making small changes toward better health. A few have even gone plant-based!

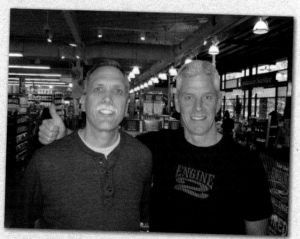

traveling

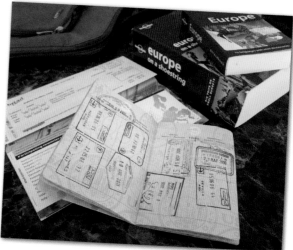

I spend most of the year living out of my suitcase. Work keeps me on the road fairly often and when I'm not traveling for work, I'm traveling for pleasure—my husband, pugs, and I are sort of a new-age vagabond family. We can always make it work, and with my tips, you can, too!

Airports and gas stations are starting to offer healthier options. Even the smallest gas station or airport terminal usually has apples and bananas for sale. Many more are selling hummus, oatmeal (just add hot water), peanuts or trail mix, fresh salads, and snack bars that are "accidentally" vegan.

I've also been pleasantly surprised by the snack options on many airlines. Many of the complimentary snacks

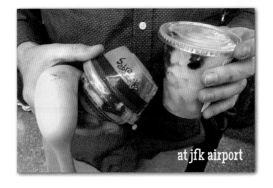

at jfk airport

are vegan, but even the snack boxes for sale on board usually have at least one vegan option. I flew a smaller airline recently and was delighted to see they were selling Dr. McDougall's Right Foods oatmeal!

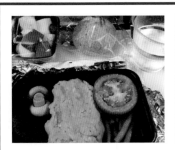 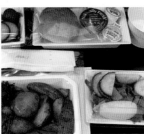

Most airlines, especially if you are traveling internationally, offer a vegan meal option if you call ahead.

Traveling with My Pressure Cooker

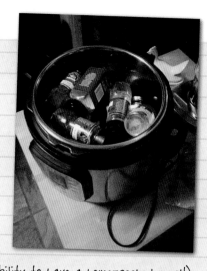

When traveling by car, I always take my pressure cooker for a makeshift hotel "stove." Not only can you cook up beans, grains, or potatoes quickly, most pressure cookers also have a sauté setting (which operates the same way as a skillet on the stove) as well as a slow-cooker feature. It's a great way to stay plant-based (and on a budget!) while traveling. (Since I travel near full-time, often staying in hotels for weeks on end, I love the ability to have a home-cooked meal!)

Along with my pressure cooker, I pack my most-used spices (in plastic snack bags) and store them in the pressure cooker along with a measuring spoon and cup to use the space. I also take a hand-operated can opener, a serving spoon, a small spatula, a knife, a small cutting board, and a reusable bowl, plate, and spork. (If you don't want to take a knife and cutting board, you can precut your veggies or buy precut vegetables, minced garlic, and diced onion.)

I love making steel-cut oats or tofu scramble for breakfast. I'm also fond of making my chilis and soups in my cooker. A super-easy chili is a can of black beans, a can of kidney beans (both drained and rinsed), a can of diced tomatoes (preferably with added flavor like jalapeños, or fire-roasted), a chili seasoning packet, and a can or two of water or broth (refill one of your cans). Let it warm/slow-cook all day!

Of course it's always healthier (and cheaper) to bring your own snacks, but it's comforting to know you still have some kind of choice if you forgot.

plant-based travel foods—what to pack

Unless otherwise noted, the following packaged foods are ready to eat. A few require microwave cooking or hot water, but most hotel rooms come equipped with a coffeepot so you can make hot water. Any gas station or coffee shop will also have hot water, and flight attendants also have hot water—just ask!

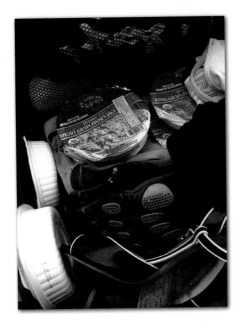

For more information, see "How to Travel on a Plant-Based Diet (What to Pack, Snacks, and More!)" on my blog, HappyHerbivore.com/blog.[i] You can also check out other travel posts and tips by clicking the "Travel" icon under Topics.

When writing this book, I tried to find every option available. I haven't personally tried every item noted here, but wanted my lists to be as comprehensive as possible. All of these items should be available in the United States (through online or mail order if they're not available locally), but I can't vouch for their availability outside of the United States.

OIL-FREE PLANT-BASED TRAVEL FOODS

Products change, so do check the ingredients list to be sure that the item is still oil-free.

» homemade Happy Herbivore muffins and granola bars (see my cookbooks or website).

» Dr. McDougall's Right Foods: Dr. McDougall makes a number of soups, oatmeals, lentil dishes, pilafs, muesli, and noodle bowls that come in a cup (add hot water). He also has a line of ready-made soups in Tetra Paks (no water necessary). You can't take them in your carry-on, but they're great in a suitcase.

» Eden Organics canned Cajun Rice & Beans, Brown Rice & Green Lentils, Caribbean Rice & Beans, and other flavors

» precooked quinoa: Minsley, GoGo, or generic

» precooked rice: Minsley, GoGo, Lundberg, or generic (microwave)

» Minsley precooked oatmeal (microwave)

» instant oatmeal packets (add hot water)

» shelf-stable tofu: Mori-Nu, Trader Joe's brand

---

i. See http://happyherbivore.com/2012/11/how-travel-plant-based-diet-pack-snacks/.

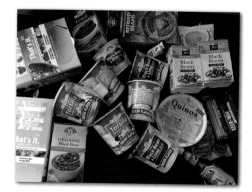

- » refried bean mix: Mother Earth, Taste Adventures, Santa Fe Bean Company (add hot water)
- » Casbah hummus mix—also great sprinkled on a salad! (add water)
- » individual packets of peanut butter
- » That's It fruit bars
- » soy milk powder
- » California Suncakes
- » beans in Tetra Paks (sold at Whole Foods Market)
- » Fantastic World Foods Tofu Scrambler mix (add tofu)
- » freeze-dried or air-dried fruits and vegetables: Mother Earth, Harmony House Foods, Just Fruit, Just Veggies, North Bay Trading Co.
- » NuturMe baby food
- » nondairy milk in aseptic cartons: Pure Almond, Silk, and other brands
- » falafel mix: Orgran (gluten-free), Near East
- » mac and cheese: Road's End Organics (gluten-free option) (boil in a coffeepot; *see Coffeepot Pasta sidebar*)
- » couscous (add hot water)
- » Lärabars raw, dried-fruit-and-nut bars
- » condiments: I carry a small spray bottle of Bragg Liquid Aminos (it makes for a great dressing paired with fresh lemon juice) and a small bottle of Cholula hot sauce. You can also buy soy sauce and tamari in packets, or save up the ones you get when you buy vegetable sushi. Recently I've found packets of Cholula and Sriracha as well.

VEGAN (BUT NOT OIL-FREE) TRAVEL FOODS

- » Fantastic World Foods hummus mix, Tabouli Salad (add tomato), falafel (add hot water), sloppy joe (add tomato paste), vegetarian chili (add beans, tomatoes, and hot water), taco filling (add hot water), Nature's Burger (add hot water), instant black beans (add hot water), refried beans (add hot water)
- » Wild Garden premade hummus
- » Santa Fe Bean Company instant refried beans
- » Casbah Tabouli (add tomato)

- » GoPicnic ready-to-eat meals: several vegan options
- » Eden Organics canned beans and rice (many flavors)
- » Food for Lovers Vegan Queso
- » Nacheeze nacho-style "cheese"
- » Worthington canned vegetarian meats: ground burger, franks, Diced Chik ("chicken"), and more
- » "meal" bars: Clif Bar, Luna Bar, ProBar, and others
- » Primal Strips meatless jerky
- » Nature Valley granola bars (contains honey)
- » BelVita breakfast biscuits
- » Fritos Bean Dip, and 7-Eleven's generic brand for canned bean dip
- » Erin Baker's Breakfast Cookies: a few varieties are vegan

supermarkets and fruit stands

Don't forget these exist when you're traveling. You can stop at supermarkets and load up on the salad bar or premade foods from the deli, or on healthful choices from the produce section or packaged-food aisles. When traveling abroad I make great use of the local markets and stands. One of the best snacks I ever had was a mango on a stick cut into the shape of a flower in Mexico. I also nabbed roasted corn on the cob with lime juice.

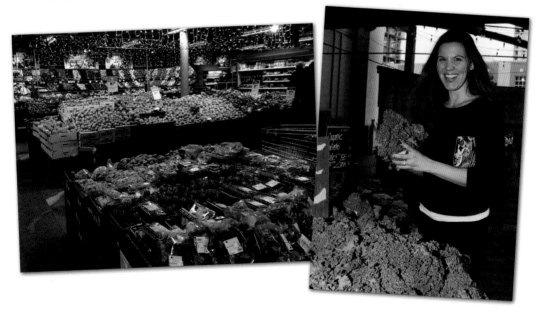

best bets at roadside restaurant chains

These items are subject to change; check the restaurant's website for up-to-date information.

Au Bon Pain: bagels, soups, salads, sandwiches

Chili's: salad, tortilla with beans, steamed vegetables

Chipotle: vegetarian burrito, veggie fajitas without cheese; tofu Sofritas

Cibo Express (airports): always changing, but multiple vegan options

Denny's: veggie burger, baked potato, oatmeal, skillets

Gas stations: Fritos bean dip, most pretzels, oatmeal, fresh fruit and vegetables

Jack in the Box: tortilla bowl, sesame bread sticks, pita bread, salad

Jason's Deli: vegetarian vegetable soup, Mediterranean wrap

Johnny Rockets: Streamliner burger (order without butter on bun)

KFC: three-bean salad, side salad

Long John Silver's: salad, rice

McDonald's: plain bagel with jelly, oatmeal

Starbucks: oatmeal, fruit/veg plates

Subway: salads, veggie subs, apple slices

Taco Bell: bean burritos (or substitute beans for meat in any dish)

websites and apps

Before a trip or while I'm on the road, I'm a huge fan of simply Googling, say, "vegan + Montreal" to see what I find. You can also look on HappyCow.net.

If you have an iPhone, try the VeganXpress app, a guide to what's vegan at popular restaurant and fast-food chains. The HappyCow VeginOut app for Android lists vegan and vegetarian restaurants worldwide. Also check out my book *Vegan in Europe*.

Coffeepot Pasta

My cousin Missy lived in a very strict dorm. She wasn't allowed any kind of appliance in her room except a coffeepot. A testament to her genius, Missy learned how to cook spaghetti in her coffeepot. To make pasta in a coffeepot, fill it with water to the max (don't bother with a filter) and put your pasta in the coffeepot. The pot will fill with very hot water and, assuming it has a built-in hot plate, it will stay hot. Let it hang out and cook until it's soft.

hotels (and dorms)

Whenever I can, I try to stay in hotels that have kitchenettes so I can prepare my meals at least some of the time. It's not only healthier, but it's more economical, and after a few days, I tire of "eating out."

My "away from home" meals aren't necessarily elaborate—oatmeal, tofu scramble, beans and rice with salsa, burritos and hummus wraps, salads, soups, baked potatoes. (I'm on vacation after all!) But I enjoy "eating in" during our trips.

If I can't rent a room with a kitchenette I try to pack my electric pressure cooker (*see Traveling with My Pressure Cooker box*) so I can make kale, vegetables (like potatoes or corn), chilis, and soups on demand.

If your hotel room has a coffeemaker (most do) you can also heat up water to make oatmeal, one of Dr. McDougall's Right Foods (and many of the other options on the Plant-Based Travel Foods list)—or pasta. (You heard me!)

camping and backpacking

At most campgrounds you will have access to a grill, either at your own site or in a communal area, and with a grill you can make pretty much anything you would at home on a stove with a pot or skillet. The same is true for those portable gas camp stoves. (I often use one in my cooking demos!)

If you want easy fare that doesn't require much (if any) cooking, *consult the Plant-Based Travel Foods list* and also consider bringing canned soups, canned beans and refried beans, canned vegetables, and a small jar of salsa. And don't forget nondairy milk, which comes in individual servings the size of a juice box!

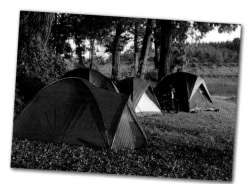

One of my favorite simple meals is canned beans with precooked quinoa and salsa. I use flavored salsas like peach and mango to keep it interesting.

CAMPFIRE MAKE-AHEAD MEALS

Muffins travel beautifully, and no one is going to turn down cupcakes or cookies at a campsite either! You can also make bean or veggie burgers ahead of time and keep them in your cooler. Frozen commercial meat and cheese substitutes will also keep in a cooler.

For easy soup and chili prep, put all the spices together in a labeled bag so you just dump the contents and go. I've also mixed together the seasonings for tofu scramble with shelf-stable tofu and, just before eating, added fresh cilantro and tomato and loaded it into tortillas.

FOOD SAFETY

Most whole (uncut) vegetables and fruits hold up well without refrigeration, and the rest will stay fresh in a cooler.

KEEP COOL: berries, leafy greens (spinach/lettuce), celery, cucumbers, pickles (once opened)

ROOM TEMP: avocados, melons, peaches, nectarines, plums, apples, pears, bananas, tomatoes, onions, garlic, potatoes, mangoes, winter squashes, peppers, pineapple, jalapeños

FREEZE-DRIED MEALS

The following companies make vegan options: Outdoor Herbivore, Mountain House, Harmony House Foods, Backpacker's Pantry, MaryJanesFarm, and AlpineAire. You can find them online and at outdoor recreational stores like R.E.I.

FOIL PACKS

To make a foil pack, tear off a long piece of heavy-duty foil. Place food such as veggies, fruits, mushrooms, or tofu in the middle, and add seasonings and an ice cube (omit if you have wet veggies like squash or onions). Bring the two long sides together and fold foil over the food. Fold over three or four more times, then fold and crimp remaining sides. (It should look like a square.) Place on hot coals and cook, turning every so often if you can, but don't touch foil with your hands—it's hot! Cook time depends on your ingredients, but roughly ten to twenty minutes. If your meal is not finished, wrap it back up and toss it back on the coals.

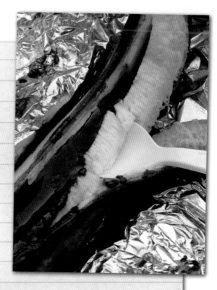

Two Essential Camping Recipes

BANANA BOATS

1. Place each banana on a 12-inch square of foil; crimp and shape so they sit flat.
2. Cut each banana lengthwise ½ inch deep, leaving ½ inch uncut at both ends. Pull each banana peel open, forming a pocket. Fill pockets with chocolate chips.
3. Grill bananas, over medium heat for 4 to 5 minutes.

S'MORES

Follow the same recipe as for the banana boats, except substitute vegan marshmallows for bananas.

GRILLED FARE

Grilled vegetables are awesome, and most campsites are equipped with a grill—just remember to bring your own tongs and plates! Grilled veggies, fruit kabobs, and skewered tofu (grilled and with peanut sauce) are where it's at!

things to grill

potatoes
red bell peppers
mushrooms
eggplant
beets
squash (any, especially yellow summer squash)
onions
corn (add chili powder and lime juice—trust me!)
carrots

pineapple
pears
peaches
apples
tofu
asparagus (squeeze lemon juice on it!)
jalapeños
romaine lettuce
vegan hot dogs
(okay, not a vegetable, I admit)

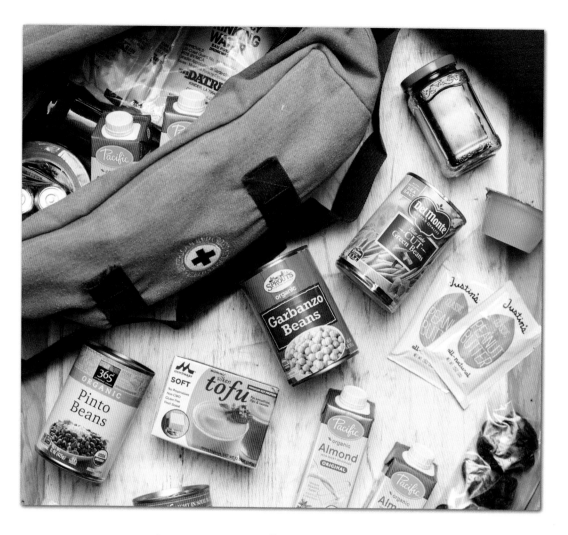

vegan travel emergency kit

In addition to the basics (matches, first aid supplies, blankets in cold climates, etc.), here are a few items to keep on hand in case disaster strikes: canned beans and vegetables (plus a hand-crank can opener), peanut butter, shelf-stable crackers, dried fruits, shelf-stable tofu, individual boxes of soy milk, ready-to-eat cereal, applesauce, and fruit cups. (*For more ideas, see earlier parts of the Traveling section.*) Don't forget about pet food!

For more information and a sample emergency menu, see "Disaster Planning for Vegetarians" on the Vegetarian Resource Group website.

TEBBEN: PLANT-BASED SOLDIER
(july 2013)

HH: What inspired you to adopt a plant-based diet?

I started out learning about the nutritional benefits of reducing meat consumption. Both cancer and heart disease run in my family, and I wanted to find a way to mitigate the risk of future medical issues. It didn't take long for me to learn about the ethical realities of consuming animal products. That is when I dropped eggs and dairy from my diet. As I've learned more about the food industry, I've also come to understand the overarching global sustainability issues of factory farming and excessive meat consumption.

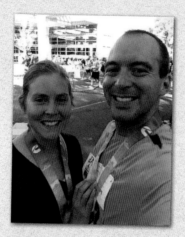

have to work out as much to maintain the same level of fitness. During my first two years of being plant-based, I reached a very healthy weight, and I haven't fluctuated more than a pound or two, regardless of changes in my workout habits. Obviously I have to eat more calories when I am working out harder and more often, but I always eat until I'm full.

HH: What kind of benefits have you experienced since your transition to a plant-based lifestyle?

Shortly after that transition, I began to feel better overall. I found that I don't

I don't count calories or carbs. I just make good choices on types of foods. I eat mostly vegetables, plus a good variety of fruits, nuts/seeds, and whole (preferably sprouted) grains. I even change up my milk choices between almond, hemp, soy, flax, and coconut.

A plant-based diet also makes it easy to avoid the pitfalls of fast food. Few places have good veggie options, and even by meat-eater standards, most of that stuff is unhealthy. I can grab an awesome premade or assemble-yourself salad at a grocery store and just skip the burger joint for about the same price.

HH: Can you tell us about your experience being plant-based in the Army? You mentioned that it can be difficult at times and that you have to be practical in certain situations. How do you make it work?

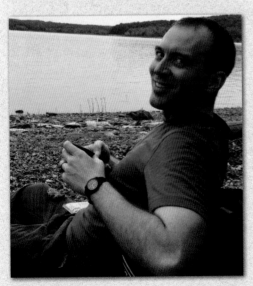

When facing a situation that would go against my plant-based lifestyle, I consider the situation and my resources and identify my options. I evaluate each option on its feasibility and acceptability, and I make my decision.

Some decisions I have very little control over. My boots, for example, are required by regulation to be made of leather. The

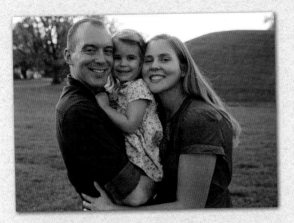

Army regulation governing uniforms (DA PAM 670–1) states that combat boots will be made of "tan-colored, flesh-side-out cattlehide leather." Even if a vegan combat boot existed, it would be out of regulation. As a result, I've worn my last pair of boots for almost four years, and finally had to break down and buy a new pair.

During certain training or deployed operations, we are required to eat Meals Ready to Eat (MREs). While I always grab one of the vegetarian MREs, I know that they will likely contain egg or dairy products. While it is very important to me to remain plant-based, it is imperative that I fulfill my obligations. I joined knowing that I would not always have my first choice in some matters.

The Army has made significant strides in supporting its soldiers. In Iraq in 2011, our dining facility had a decently stocked salad bar every day, and "vegetarian bar" a couple times a week. It usually consisted of bean and cheese burritos, or a pan of boiled lima beans (sometimes with cubed ham?!?), but at least they made an effort. Soy milk was also available in very limited supply.

HH: Have you experienced any other obstacles? What was your transition like?

The biggest hurdle I've encountered since I decided to go plant-based has been finding time to invest in healthy eating. It is really quick and easy to microwave a frozen dinner, or throw a chicken breast on the grill, but just a few extra minutes of prep time to make a salad or some quinoa is a huge investment in your health and the future of the planet.

The best part about eating a plant-based diet is discovering new foods and dishes that you may have never come across. I still miss certain things, but I can almost always find a plant-based alternative. I'm still working on finding a replacement for Mom's meatloaf, though.

HH: Do you have any advice for others who are new to or looking to try a plant-based diet?

This is by far the best way to get and stay healthy. Being vegan forces you to avoid a lot of the greasy fast food that you probably want to avoid anyway. That being said, ease into it. Set achievable goals, such as:

» No fast-food burgers, but burgers at home are okay occasionally.
» Designate only a night or two per week that you will eat meat, then eventually cut those meals out as well.
» Progress gradually: Cut out meat, then eggs, then dairy.
» Experiment with tempeh, seitan, and tofu. They don't totally replace the "meat experience," but you can make some incredible meals with them. Use them in your favorite meat-based recipe if you start to feel nostalgic.

UPDATE (summer 2014):

We're living in Virginia now, just outside of Washington, DC. The whole family is still plant-based (almost exclusively vegan), and we try to eat locally produced whole foods as much as possible. Our son (turning two this Sunday) has a severe milk allergy, so eating a plant-based diet really helps us avoid allergic reactions. My wife has purchased several of the Happy Herbivore's 7-Day Meal Plans (http://www.getmealplans.com) that we rotate through as well.

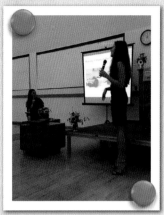

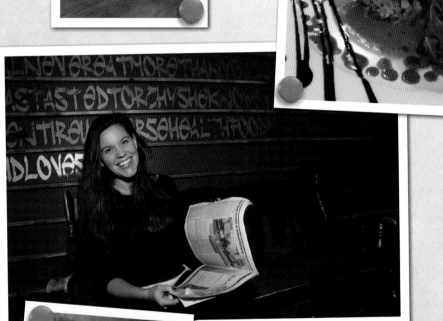

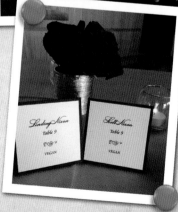

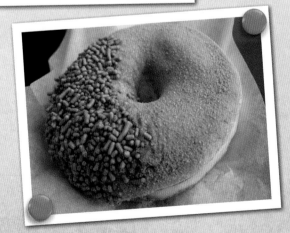

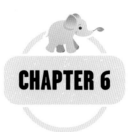

CHAPTER 6

challenges

"It's part of life to have
obstacles. It's about overcoming obstacles;
that's the key to happiness."

—HERBIE HANCOCK—

Even the best changes in life, such as getting married or having children, still bring new challenges with them, and choosing a healthier lifestyle—by adopting a plant-based diet—has its challenges as well. Food addictions, cravings, social pressure, and negativity are some of the hurdles you might face during your journey.

In this section I touch on some major challenges and provide a few tips for dealing with each in turn. Remember: The prescription for any challenge is patience, time, and perseverance.

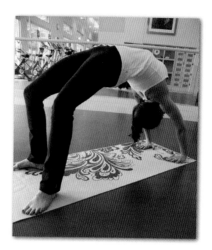

food addictions

Food addiction goes far beyond what we think of as "emotional eating." Food can be as physically addicting as a drug.

Sugar, for example, causes opioid production in the brain. (Opioids are natural chemicals that behave like manufactured opiates, such as heroin.) The release of opioids then triggers a release of dopamine—the neurotransmitter responsible for everything that feels good.[1]

Similarly, when the body breaks down casein, a milk protein and known carcinogen, casomorphins (yes, as in morphine) are created.[2] Casomorphins, like sugar, have an opioid effect on the brain, making dairy as addictive as a drug. Cheese has the *highest* concentration of casein of any food, which is why people often struggle to stop eating cheese—they're literally hooked!

We're also wired to derive pleasure from foods with lots of fat and calories. It's a built-in survival mechanism going back thousands of years, when calorie-rich foods (and foods in general) were scarce and humans were much more active.

This wiring is why ice cream, cheesecake, and brownies taste so good. They're very rich in calories (also high in both sugar and fat), and they also contain casein, which keeps us coming back for more. Even whole plant foods that are high in fat and/or rich in calories can give us that pleasure sensation. It's why people love peanut butter so much! Have you ever wondered why you can't put down that bag of potato chips? Oil is highly caloric and 100 percent fat, making it very pleasure inducing and extremely addictive.[i]

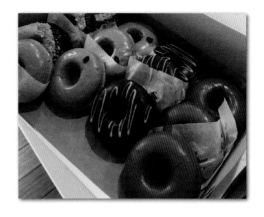

We're not weak, we're addicted, and the food manufacturers are our enablers. Modern foods are tastier than ever before, because the chemicals responsible for pleasure activation have been isolated and artificially concentrated to send us straight to what the manufactured-food industry calls a "bliss point."[ii]

For example, food scientists at the big manufacturers have fiddled with the distribution of fat globules to affect their absorption rate (or "mouthfeel" as it's known in the industry). The physical shape of salt has also been altered so it hits taste buds harder and faster, improving its "flavor burst." Sugar crystals have been manipulated in numerous ways as well to increase the allure of processed foods.

So we keep eating these foods, even when we know they're not good for us, because we can't help ourselves. They've got us: hook, line, and sinker.

breaking food addictions

The only way to break a food addiction (or a food habit) is the way you break *any* addiction: abstinence. You have to stop eating those foods—stop getting high on dairy and sugar. Break the cycle! It's not going to be a picnic, but your health is worth it. Plus if you start eating only healthy foods, you will begin to *crave* only

---

i. Our intense love of processed foods may be what Dr. David A. Kessler, former administrative director of the Food and Drug Administration, calls "conditioned hypereating" in his 2009 book, *The End of Overeating.*

ii. The bliss point refers to the precise amount of sugar or fat or salt that will send consumers over the moon.

healthy foods. Fast-food and junk food cravings will become a distant memory. I've seen it a hundred times with my clients—and myself.

It's not uncommon to experience withdrawal and detox symptoms like headache or fatigue when breaking a food addiction and/or transitioning to a plant-based diet. To make it as pain-free as possible, be sure to drink plenty of water and get plenty of rest. Most important, stick with it—it will get better.

BREAKING SUGAR

Use fruit instead of sugar. For example, in my 7-Day Meal Plans (http://www.getmealplans.com) oatmeal is frequently sweetened with unsweetened applesauce instead of sugar, or mixed with lots of fruits such as frozen berries or fresh banana slices.

If you must use sugar, sprinkle a tiny bit on top—just enough to make it palatable. (And keep reducing it—the amount you feel you need should decrease over time.)

Nibble on frozen fruits, one at a time, if your sweet tooth is calling. If you're dying for ice cream, send two frozen bananas with a little cinnamon and almond or soy milk through your food processor to make banana "ice cream." You can also eat sweet potatoes with cinnamon for a sweet snack. If you opt for dried fruits, make sure no sugar, oil, or juice has been added.

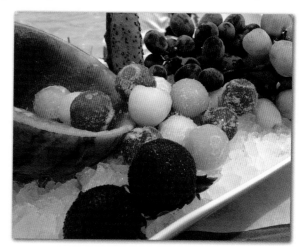

A note about sweeteners: I'm of the opinion that sugar is sugar. While some sweeteners, like pure maple syrup or sucanat, are a touch more nutritious and less processed than white sugar, they're still sweeteners, and should be used sparingly. That said, I do make plant-based cookies, cupcakes, and muffins from time to time—I love a good treat! And I'll use a little bit of raw sugar or maple syrup when I do, but otherwise, I've really cut back on my consumption.

BREAKING DAIRY

Find suitable dairy substitutes if you need to—homemade or commercial. My cookbooks include many vegan "cheese" recipes, but you can also find recipes online or try those in *The Ultimate Uncheese Cookbook* by Jo Stepaniak and *Artisan Vegan Cheese* by Miyoko Schinner. More and more commercial substitutes—for milk, cream, butter, yogurt, whipped cream, and all types of cheeses—are available every day; look for them at your local health food store. *See "Vegan (Not Plant-Based) Substitutes: Meat, Cheese, Ice Cream, and More" in chapter four for a list.*

If you miss the creamy texture of cheese, sour cream, or yogurt, try using other foods with a similar consistency, such as avocado, cashew cream (blend soaked cashew nuts with water), walnuts (blend with other items, like kale, and a bit of water or broth, to make a butter), and hummus.

BREAKING SALT

Instead of turning to salt for flavor, ramp up the spices and herbs already used in the dish. Alternatively, use commercial salt-free seasonings. The brand Mrs. Dash has several interesting, flavor-packed spice blends that are sodium-free. (My personal favorites are Fiesta Lime and Southwest Chipotle.) Spike is another brand with many salt-free seasoning options. Maine Coast Sea Vegetables' Sea Seasonings kelp and dulse granules are another option. The popular salt brand Morton makes a salt-free salt substitute as well, though it is made with potassium chloride, which may not be safe for some patients with certain preexisting medical conditions (talk to your doctor).

BREAKING FAT

Unlike dairy, sugar, and salt, fat is a bit trickier to replace in terms of mouthfeel because you won't find that rich "fat" taste in other foods. You can, however, find lower-fat options that have similar textures.

Instead of frying, bake. You'll still get a nice, dense crispness, especially if you broil briefly at the end. If you love crunchy nuts as a snack, try baking chickpeas with spices as a healthier, low-fat alternative.

To replace mayonnaise, blend 12 ounces of soft or silken tofu (such as Mori-Nu) with 2 to 3 tablespoons Dijon mustard, 2 teaspoons distilled white vinegar, plus agave nectar (or honey) and fresh lemon juice to taste.

AMI: FORMER LOW-CARBER AND EX—CHEESE ADDICT
february 2013

HH: You initially found your way to a vegetarian diet thanks to your husband. Can you tell us a little more about that?

When I met my husband in 2009, he had been a vegetarian for five years. He was also an amazing cook, so I tried being a vegetarian. We even had a vegetarian wedding reception, complete with vegan cupcakes at our wedding.

HH: What were your health and diet like before you met your husband?

Prior to meeting my husband, I had been a low-carber trying desperately to maintain an 87-pound weight loss for the previous three years. Attempting to maintain my weight was really tough; I gained back half the weight I had lost before I even met my husband. I weighed 210 pounds back in 2004. Weight had always been an issue for me, and my cholesterol was 242.

HH: I find a lot of people assume a vegetarian diet is automatically healthy, but that's not always the case. I've met a number of people who were vegetarian or vegan but were still overweight, sick, etc., because they weren't keeping the "veg" in vegan or vegetarian, as I say. What kind of vegetarian diet did you eat? And what spawned your dietary change to a whole food, plant-based diet?

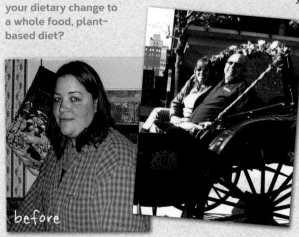

before

We loved to eat! We ate a lot of dairy and high-fat foods. But our busy lives, stress, career changes for both of us, and everyday life began to take a toll on our health. Our clothes didn't fit, and we had to do something. I bought Brendan Brazier's book *Thrive*. I read it cover to cover and attempted a couple of recipes. Then it sat collecting dust because I wasn't ready.

The following year, we tried Dr. Barnard's 21-Day Vegan Kickstart. It worked, but we fell off the wagon in Chicago. Foiled by Gino's East Pizza!

At my annual checkup my cholesterol scores were: 229 total; 177 triglycerides; 52 HDL cholesterol; and 142 LDL cholesterol.

During that time, I purchased Dr. Caldwell B. Esselstyn's book, *Prevent and Reverse Heart Disease*. I read it cover to cover, made a couple of recipes, and then Dr. Esselstyn sat on the bookshelf next to Brendan Brazier, shaking his head in disappointment.

Spring came last year, and found us at our heaviest in years. That's when I bought *The Happy Herbivore Cookbook*. I remarked to my husband, Bill, that this I can do! I can eat this way and be happy! I'm a sucker for cookbooks with photos!

Everything looked amazing and it was just the push I needed. I bought *The Engine 2 Diet* by Rip Esselstyn shortly thereafter. I was building a compendium of information and recipes to sustain us. I was trying to figure out how to commit to a whole food, plant-based diet. A few months later, I stumbled upon *Forks Over Knives* on Netflix. That's it. Yes!!!

And we are doing it! On December 27, 2011, we got down to business. Several false starts, excuses, and laziness prevented us from getting started earlier, because we had the tools all along. However, those tools sat there collecting dust and waiting for us to get smart and get busy.

HH: Did you gradually cut out the dairy, etc., or did you jump straight in?

We jumped in cold turkey, we got our behinds to the gym, found fitness that is fun for us, and learned a lot about ingredients and what we are really capable of accomplishing. I love being a recipe scientist and constructing meals that we truly enjoy and that nurture us. I attended the Farms2Forks Immersion Weekend in Austin, Texas, to learn even more about how we could thrive. I learned so much from the Farms2Forks team over the course of the weekend. I came home rejuvenated and focused on making this change a permanent one and helping others to do so as well. I wanted to be a plant-based food coach for my friends and family.

HH: Did you lose any weight?

I have lost 45 pounds, so many inches, and gained a bunch of muscle, but most of all, I gained the empowerment of knowing I can sustain this lifestyle. My cholesterol score after six months of plant-based living: 139 total; 91 triglycerides; 40 HDL cholesterol; and 81 LDL cholesterol. Almost a 50 percent reduction! I take no meds and feel amazing!

I *love* my whole food, plant-based lifestyle. It has made a tremendous difference in my health, my energy level,

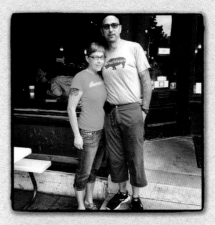

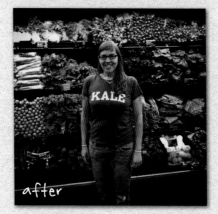

after

and my relationship with food. My husband's, too! He's lost 73 pounds.

HH: With your weight in check and you feeling so good, what are your goals and focus now?

I am focused now on continuing to improve my fitness level with strength training, running, swimming, and yoga. My whole life has improved since making this change. I've been certified in Plant-Based Nutrition through the T. Colin Campbell Foundation/eCornell. I have also become a Fitness Nutrition specialist through the National Academy of Sports Medicine. I am part of the Engine 2 Extra team, and I help others on a daily basis with their plant-based journey.

UPDATE (summer 2014):

Since becoming plant-strong, my husband and I have continued to share our passion for healthy food with young athletes in the USA Boxing program. In spring 2014, we opened our own nonprofit youth boxing program, where we teach about fitness, boxing, and plant-based nutrition. We also provide healthy snacks to the kids each day. Teaching the kids to seek out better choices for snacks and meals is the foundation to them having a healthy and strong body. We also have plans for a series of budget-minded plant-based cooking classes so the kids can learn how easy it is to make plant-based meals at home on a budget.

To replace sour cream, blend 12 ounces of soft or silken tofu (such as Mori-Nu) with 2 to 4 tablespoons lemon juice, ½ teaspoon distilled white vinegar, 1 teaspoon dry mustard powder, a dash of garlic powder, and agave nectar (or honey) to taste.

If you can't have soy, search for recipes for vegan mayo or sour cream using cashews as a base instead of tofu.

On sandwiches, hummus or guacamole is a great substitute for mayo—ditto when trying to replace cream cheese on a bagel.

For additional tips on how to cook and bake without oil and fat, see chapter eight. For a list of books about food addiction, see the Appendix, "Learn More about Plant-Based Living."

a note about cravings

A question I often hear is, "I'm craving meat [or cheese]; shouldn't I listen to my body and eat what it wants?" The idea that the body is telling us what we need with cravings is lovely in theory, but not true in reality. As stated earlier in this chapter, dairy, for example, is as addictive as a drug, so your body (and mind) will physically crave it once you've stopped eating it. In other words, you're going through withdrawal. Here's another way to think about it: When smokers are craving a cigarette, should they listen to their bodies and have a smoke? Cravings for foods will pass in time, especially if you stop thinking about them as "food," or options. (And if I "listened to my body," I'd subsist on chocolate and cupcakes!)

Dr. David A. Kessler, a former Food and Drug Administration director, says educating ourselves about food can help us alter our perceptions about what types of food are desirable—that we can undergo "perceptual shifts" about large portion sizes and processed foods. For example, Dr. Kessler notes that when people who once loved to eat steak become vegetarians, they typically begin to view animal protein as disgusting, just as past smokers who now find cigarettes or their smell repulsive.[3]

This has certainly proved true in my life. The smell of grease and greasy foods now makes me queasy, even though there was a period of my life where I ate French fries almost every day. And if I never smell fried calamari again, it won't be a day too soon.

My dad also had his own experience at Thanksgiving the year after he went plant-based, and *you can read his story in "Common Objections" in chapter four.*

THE PSYCHOLOGICAL NATURE OF CRAVINGS

We associate foods with happy memories of holidays and family traditions (e.g., Thanksgiving and Christmas), times when we experienced comfort or love ("Mom used to make this for me when I was sick"), and happy times in our lives ("I used to make these cookies for my roommates in college"). Food can also be part of our cultural heritage and identity ("I'm Italian"), and so we worry that without these foods we'll be missing a part of ourselves.

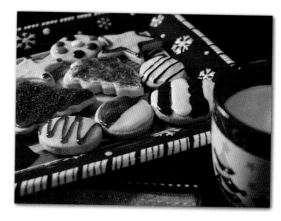

From these associations, foods can evoke certain feelings in us, and when we're having a hard time or a bad day, we turn to foods that make us feel good—and often those foods contain an ingredient with an opioid effect, too! In other words, eating sometimes becomes a form of self-soothing. (Emotional hunger is sudden, while physical hunger is gradual.)

Whenever a craving hits—whether biological or psychological—here is something to remember: **If hunger is not the problem, food is not the solution.** Taking a moment to really think about and examine your cravings can help you overcome them. Also try saying, out loud, "I'm not hungry, but I'm going to eat this anyway," or, "I know this is not a healthful choice and I'm going to eat it anyway," and be dazzled by how effective this is at steering you in the right direction.

I find the out-loud affirmation incredibly difficult to do, even when I'm home alone and no one is there to hear me or judge me—not even my dogs! That's good, though, because then I don't eat junk food. (I also find that it's when I'm alone that all those cravings start bubbling up. A coincidence? I think not.)

tasteless taste buds

As we've seen, processed foods are loaded with salt, oil, and sugar (aptly abbreviated SOS)—a killer combo for making food super addictive. The more sugar, oil, or salt you eat, the more you crave it. But the "foods" filled with these substances have another adverse effect: They rob you of experiencing flavor.

Oil coats your tongue, so it's a little like eating with a glove on. Meanwhile, salt and sugar over-stimulate the taste buds, which damages your taste receptors. The more salt, sugar, and oil you eat, the more salt, sugar, and oil your food will need to taste "good"—it's a vicious cycle!

Luckily, you can heal your taste buds! How? By eating a plant-based diet free from processed foods. *The Pleasure Trap* authors Douglas J. Lisle and Alan Goldhamer agree. They call processed foods "magic foods," and say the way to break their spell is to avoid them. Food may taste bland for a few weeks, but soon (within a

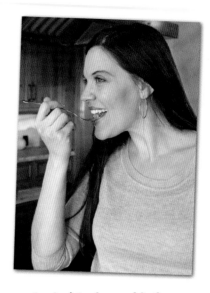

few months at most) you'll have healthy, sensitive taste buds.[4] And a world of taste will open up to you, as you develop the ability to discern more subtle flavors!

negativity

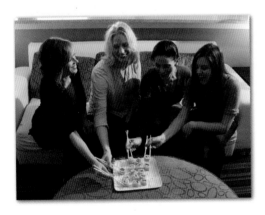

When I first adopted a plant-based diet, I assumed there would be some teasing and mockery from my friends, some peer pressure trying to get me to "cheat," and perhaps a few questions or concerns. But what I *never* expected was the open hostility.

Some friends were downright angry. It went well beyond being negative or not being supportive. It was as if my new lifestyle insulted them at their very core and as if I had deeply offended them by putting plants on my plate.

There were many painful moments. One friend said, immediately, "Well, I guess we can't hang out anymore." Another kept canceling dinner plans, and after

MICHELLE: OVERCAME AN EATING DISORDER
october 2012

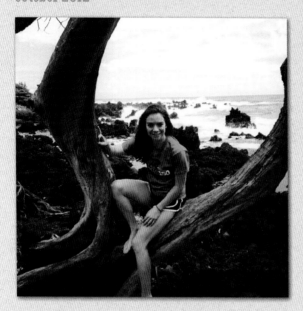

HH: You were diagnosed with an eating disorder a few years ago. Can you tell us a little bit about that and its role (if any) with your transition to a plant-based diet?

Ever since my father's second divorce nine years ago, I've been in a constant battle with my weight and body image. The excess weight began to creep on during my second-grade year due to our dependency on fast food and the lack of an immediate maternal figure (my mother lived in the area, but my father tried to keep her out of my life and my brothers' lives as much as possible).

I was taunted by my peers about my weight throughout elementary school, as well as by my new stepmother, brother, and sister. The pain was almost unbearable.

Then, by the beginning of the summer of 2010 (after I finished eighth grade), I fell into a mild depression that progressively became worse. I compensated by overexercising and consuming a thousand calories—or fewer—per day, being obsessed with keeping track of every morsel I ate, its ingredients, et cetera. The weight started coming off, although not in the healthiest manner. By the end of the summer (August), my parents realized something was wrong when they took me to get my sports physical. I was hanging in at the bottom of the healthy range for my height and weight, but was in the danger zone for being underweight and malnourished if I continued down the same path. I tried to fix the damage on my own, but my mind-set was so skewed that I had no idea where to start.

A couple months later (October 2010), I was taken to Texas Children's Hospital in the Houston Medical Center and was diagnosed with an eating disorder (the doctors never specified what it was, but I know it was a mix of anorexia and orthorexia, or "perfect eating").

HH: How did you find out about plant-based eating and why did you want to try this new lifestyle approach?

When I first ran across Happy Herbivore in May 2011, I had no intention of becoming plant-based. Simply, I was tired of eating the same boring beans and rice or salad for the meatless meals I ate at least once a day every week. Once I began preparing more meals from *The Happy Herbivore Cookbook* and your blog, I slowly began to lose interest in meat, and I spent most of my winter break researching about how to live a whole food, plant-based lifestyle, which included reading *The Engine 2 Diet*. At the turn of the new year, I gave up cow's milk and cheese, and ate significantly less fish. However, I continued to eat yogurt and seafood a few times a week to keep my parents' suspicions about another eating disorder from reappearing.

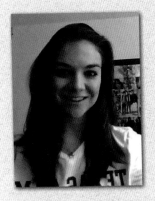

After two months of struggling to progress toward becoming 100 percent plant-based, I persuaded my mother to take me to see Rip Esselstyn speak at a Houston-area Whole Foods on February 20. After talking to Rip, I decided to not let my parents (specifically my father) halt my journey and I cut out the last culprit: my beloved nonfat Greek yogurt.

Honestly, I haven't found it too difficult to stay plant-based whatsoever. I started preparing my own meals the summer before my freshman year, so I was used to balancing homework, choir rehearsals, and track practice with cooking three meals a day.

In the evening while waiting for my dinner to cook, I would put together my sandwich or salad for lunch the next day. Another thing that has helped is keeping it simple and not trying to prepare glamorous meals unless time allowed. I always keep frozen brown rice, potatoes (sweet, white, or red), frozen vegetables, and canned low-sodium beans around in case I have a day where I'm tied up and only have ten minutes to put something together.

My friends are quite supportive and are always interested in what I bring every day for lunch. I always get comments, such as, "Your lunch looks so colorful and healthy!" or, "That salad looks great." I'm not a "pusher" for trying to get my friends to go plant-based, but from time to time, I would make Happy Herbivore muffins, cupcakes, or cookies to share on a friend's birthday (so far, I haven't had anyone *not* love a dessert I have brought.

Once we visited with a registered dietitian I had been seeing at Texas Children's Hospital to discuss going plant-based, he felt more confident that I was doing what was best for my well-being. At first, my dietitian gave the go-ahead for vegetarianism but not veganism because of possible effects of not getting enough B_{12}, such as permanent and irreversible neurological damage. I wasn't pleased with this answer, so I stuck with being plant-based but agreed to begin taking a B_{12} supplement.

My studies have become less tedious, and even though I'm not a natural athlete in any way, I've noticed several positive changes in my athletic performances as a swimmer and thrower.

Make sure that your intentions for going plant-based are in the right place. Yes, going plant-based for the environment and animal rights is a great reason, but don't do so to starve yourself and live off of vegan junk. As long as you're eating whole plant foods and staying active, you shouldn't need to worry about the way you perceive yourself. Everyone comes in all shapes and sizes and everyone is beautiful in their *own* way.

For parents' sake, educate them with as much plant-based nutrition as you can. Assure them that eating a plant-based diet is the best thing you can do for yourself, both mentally and physically. If you're an athlete, show them that there are professional athletes who are plant-based.

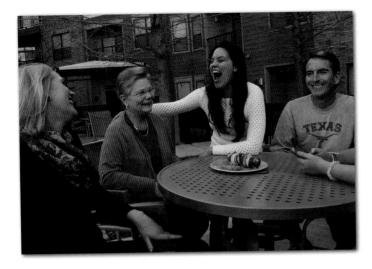

a few cancellations I asked if I had done something wrong—was she angry with me? She complained about how much I had changed and said, "Can't you go back to being the *old* Lindsay?" When I asked what she meant, she said, "The one who ate 'real' food!"

Still another friend stopped inviting me to her parties, but she still invited all of our mutual friends. When I broached the situation with her she said, "Oh, I'm not vegan. There's nothing for you to eat, so I didn't invite you." (Is that all a party is? Eating? There is no socializing?) I told her she didn't have to cater to me—she could let me worry about what I was going to eat, but I was never invited again anyway. Our friendship officially ended after she sent me a hateful e-mail saying she was going to buy meat just to throw it away to make up for all the meat I wasn't eating.

I just couldn't understand why my new lifestyle bothered my friends so much. Thankfully my story isn't entirely sad. I had many friends who were wonderfully supportive or said, "Whatever floats your boat," and those friendships only continued to blossom.

But as for the naysayers, why do some people react in such a visceral, hostile manner to someone else's choices? Author Deepak Chopra wrote, "When you feel frustrated or upset by a person or a situation, remember that you are not reacting to the person or the situation, but to your feelings about the person or the situation. These are your feelings, and your feelings are not someone else's fault."[5]

Over time, I've come up with a couple of answers that explain others' negativity and hostility toward your lifestyle and choices:

1. YOU ARE A MIRROR. Your conviction makes them reflect upon themselves, and they don't like what they see. They then attack you to make themselves feel better.

I find that when people are angry or dogmatic about something, it's always about them and their inner demons—not the person they are attacking. I like to remind myself that if they were secure with their choices (as I am with mine) they wouldn't need to attack me or my lifestyle—just as I'm not criticizing them or their choices, because that would be no better than what they're doing to me.

"I'm experimenting for right now."

2. **THERE IS COMFORT IN CONFORMITY.** Change can be unsettling—*for them*. You've just challenged the status quo. You've rocked the boat. Burst the bliss bubble. And so they feel the need to pressure you back into conformity. Don't give in, but don't argue your lifestyle, either.

"This seems to be working for me, so I'm going to stick with it for now."

Be diplomatic. A great neutralizer is "I'm experimenting for right now" or "This seems to be working for me, so I'm going to stick with it for now."

"Why is it so important to you that I try it?"

As my friend Sue once said to me so brilliantly, "Don't argue your lifestyle. Live your lifestyle. The changes in you will be enough and you won't have to open your mouth."

The desire for conformity also suggests some insecurity. Your avoidance of a food or drink that someone else loves or enjoys can make them uncomfortable. And they might feel judged for their consumption, even if you're not judging them. For example, back in college I had a friend who wasn't much of a drinker, and yet it was remarkable how often people (myself included) tried to get her to drink. "Just try this drink—you'll like it!" The question isn't why *she* wasn't drinking, but why was it so important to *me* that she have a drink? Was her abstention making me feel guilty about my own consumption? Would I feel better about my choices if she drank, too?

I once had a relative who relentlessly pressured me to eat meat by saying, "C'mon, just a bite! It won't kill you!" I finally replied, "Why is it so important to you that I try it?" My relative didn't know how to respond to that. And this person also never asked me to "just try it" again. Perhaps not my most diplomatic moment, but it *was* effective!

Remember, when people are dismissive, negative, or otherwise trying to sabotage your efforts at a healthier life, it's about them—not you.

As Deepak Chopra says, "In a world where most people are pursuing a pleasure-trapped path of self-destruction, the ability to manage being 'different' has become increasingly important... Choosing a health-promoting path may cause moments of psychological pain, moments of discomfort for which one must be prepared. With the right tools, you can improve your ability to resist social pressure."[6]

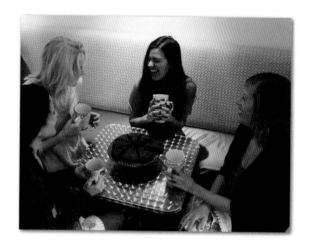

I find that most newcomers to the plant-based lifestyle are worried about their social life—specifically, how their plant-based diet is going to work socially. There's a comfort in normalcy. Who wants to be the oddball? And what do you do when you're on a date or invited to a dinner party? Or your coworkers want to go out to lunch for the boss's birthday? Or your boss buys you a Christmas ham? Or you're socializing after church and there's food? And what the heck do you tell your friends, or—gasp—MOM?

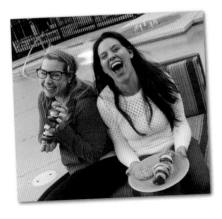

the "don't worry about me" approach

I've had friends and coworkers try to make a big deal out of my lifestyle, à la, "Oh, we can't go to lunch there because Lindsay won't find anything to eat." This usually stems from kindness and genuine concern (which I think is

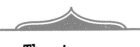

There is no way to make people like change. You can only make them feel less threatened by it.

—FREDERICK HAYES—

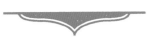

sweet and I very much appreciate), but I always tell them, "Don't worry about me. I'll find something to eat. Let's go where the group wants to go."

I can't say I've always had the most exciting meal (salad and a baked potato has happened more than once), but I've always found something to eat—and more often than not, everyone starts staring at my plate, marveling at what I've ordered, and then asks for a bite.

No one wants to feel like change is being forced on them. After seeing you change your own diet, others may feel that they have to change where they are going to eat. You've just taken their favorite steakhouse from them! You can totally neutralize that and keep it harmonious. Go with the flow. Be a great example. Make it work, and when all else fails, order a potato or a plate of broccoli and rice—and feast at home later.

There are also oodles of restaurants that go "both ways," making eating out with mixed diets a breeze! *See "Eating Out" in chapter five for ideas and suggestions.*

dinner invites

Talk to the host well in advance. I can't recommend this enough. You may think it's more considerate to keep quiet, to ensure that the host goes to no extra

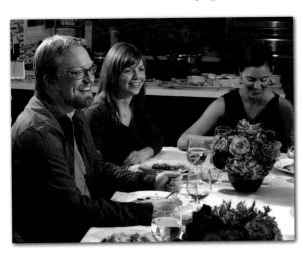

trouble. But I had a heart-breaking experience once where I said nothing at all, showed up, and the host ended up crying. She felt so bad that there was nothing for me to eat. I kept insisting it was fine, I was fine, but alas. I felt terrible for days.

When talking to the host, say something like, "I've recently switched my diet

THE HAPPY HERBIVORE GUIDE TO PLANT-BASED LIVING

and I don't want to be a burden to you, so I can bring my own meal, or something everyone can share and I can eat as my meal." (This strategy always works rather well for me.) Then I close with, "I really appreciate the invite and am looking forward to it." You can also say, "Please don't feel the need to cater to me. Please cook whatever you want to cook and were planning."

If the host insists on providing something you can eat, suggest easy options: "I love pasta. Pasta is great!" or, "Just make extra salad or vegetables for me," or even, "I love hummus!" If the host wants to make a meal that works for everyone, pasta is always a good choice because meat and cheese can be added separately. And if the host wants to make a vegan meal, well, suggest my cookbooks or website!

weddings and other catered events

With allergies being more common and specialty diets more widely recognized, I find that, more and more, event staff and caterers are either offering diet-specific options or showing a willingness to accommodate these diets in some way. It can help to call ahead or talk to the bride or groom (or event planner) to see if they can put you in touch with the food team. If nothing else, take snacks with you and eat a big meal before or after.

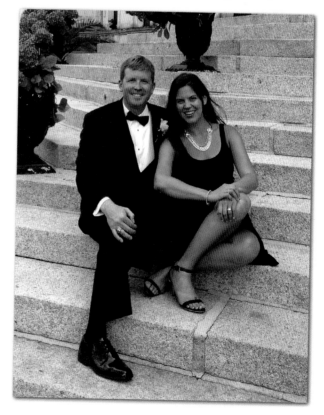

Anytime I feel strained at catered events (which is rare, because nearly all buffet lines have at least salads, crudités, and fruit to hold me over) I remind myself that I'm not there for the food.

kids' parties

When I was interviewing plant-based parents about raising plant-based kids—and specifically about how they managed birthday parties and play dates—one mom had an answer that I just loved.

"My goal is to have my daughter understand that she is not 'missing out' when it comes to food. You can miss out when it comes to playtime or watching a movie, but putting food in your body should not be the way we measure involvement in [an] activity, especially for kids."

I find most parents bring a special vegan cupcake or cookie for their kids to eat, and pack a meal and snacks for them, unless the host parent is on board with the child's dietary restrictions and will be offering plant-based options. Most parents I talk to also say they fib, especially to their children's teachers, that the kids have an *allergy* to animal products to ensure compliance.

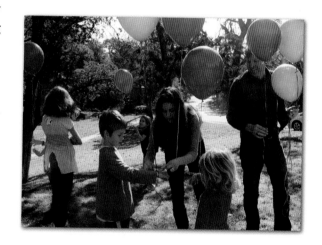

(For more information, you can also read the three-part Raising Herbies series on HappyHerbivore.com.[iii])

"but I made this for you!" (politely declining food)

One of the hardest, most soul-crushing moments for me involved a bag of Skittles. I was newly plant-based and my parents were respectful of my choice, though not yet on board. (They are now, but that's another story for another time.) My dad had returned from the gas station with a bag of Skittles—my favorite kind of Skittles, no less. My mom made a comment about how my father was having

---

iii. See http://happyherbivore.com/2013/05/how-to-raise-vegan-vegetarian-kids/; links to Parts 2 and 3 are at the bottom of this post.

iv. Back then Skittles contained gelatin, an animal by-product. They no longer do.

trouble dealing with the fact that I was grown up, which was heartbreaking (and heart melting—I'm a daddy's girl) all on its own. But then when he handed them to me I had to say, "Oh, I can't have those," and watch his smile dissolve.[iv] I could cry just thinking about it.

The saddest part was that my dad had tried to be considerate of my diet. He wanted to get me a treat and knew milk chocolates (keyword "milk") weren't an option, and he thought Skittles were a safe bet. He was crushed. And now I was crushed that he was crushed.

(In retrospect, maybe the better thing would have been to thank him, say I'd save them for later, and then discreetly discard them or give them away—but alas, hindsight.)

I've also dealt with the sad faces of loved ones who have made me something I once loved, but no longer eat; and the good-intentioned relatives who say, for example, "I scooped the chicken out of the soup for you so it's vegetarian!"

It's gotten a lot better, especially now that my husband, parents, and most of my husband's family are on board. Now, our extended families just let us do our own thing. We make our own food—and usually prepare more than enough so the curious can try some. No more sad faces or confusion.

I must also applaud my family, because they really do try. I was so touched when I showed up for a family barbecue and they'd picked up a box of vegan burgers *and* had

The Mixed-Diet Hostess

My friend Jane navigates the mixed-diet dinner party beautifully. On one occasion, she prepared a vegan pasta dish with lots of veggies as the main course, but she also had a plate of grilled chicken and a plate of cheese on the table so the vegetarians and meat eaters at the table could add their animal products of choice.

Another time, she had everyone over for brunch. She used a vegan pancake recipe, and also tweaked her muffins to be vegan. Eggs and cheese were served as well, along with sausages (both vegan and meat) and a fruit salad. It was a terrific brunch and everyone was happy.

the forethought to put foil down on the grill to prevent "cross-contamination." I'm not sure they knew how much that meant to me.

Here are some ways you can deal with this inevitable situation. All of these won't work all of the time, but you should have a few good options for any given situation.

Personally, I find saying, "Oh gosh, I just ate and I'm stuffed!" is fairly universal. You can also say something like, "Thank you for thinking of me, that is so sweet and it looks really good! I've been trying to eat healthier and I'm doing pretty well. I don't have the greatest self-control so if I let myself get off track I'll have trouble getting back on."

I asked my fans on Facebook to help out with this one, too. Here are some of my favorite responses:

"I say I have allergies. It doesn't offend people."

—BREE L.

"I thank them for the effort, but briefly explain that if I eat [identify a specific ingredient] it does not agree with me, and then I thank them again."

—REBECCA A.

"I am always honest and tell them thanks but no thanks, I don't eat [whatever's being offered]. I don't feel the need to offer up any excuses."

—DARLENE P.

"If it is a prepackaged gift, I smile, accept it, then give it to someone who is not plant-based."

—SANDRA M.

"I politely state that I don't eat [it and that]
I know my lifestyle isn't right for everyone, and not to
be upset, I will just grab a salad on my way home."

—SANDRA M.

"I say I'm [following] doctor's orders...
Strangely, people are less offended when they think
it's not by my own choice."

—DEBORAH W.

people-pleasing pitfalls (and standing your ground)

One of my fans gave this advice to a new Herbie and it's spot on:

"As long as you give in, compromise, or do anything contrary to what you are saying you believe, you are just reinforcing the idea that you are not really serious about this and can easily be swayed or bullied into what they want you to do. Just be kind, but firm. Do not budge one inch or you will never be taken seriously and the harassment will never stop."

I can attest to this with my clients. Caving to keep the peace or to please someone else nearly always backfires and you're the one who suffers. I've never had a client who succumbed to peer pressure come back saying, "That was great! I'm so glad I did that!"

Most times they were disappointed with themselves, which we could work through, but another stickier problem remained: The problem wasn't within themselves but with *other people*—those who made them cave. And once you cave to peer pressure, it's assumed you always will. If you resist after giving in once, the peer pressure intensifies, seeking your new breaking point.

I tell my clients, it's like pulling off a Band-Aid. Just pull it off. Deal with the sting all at once and get it out of the way so you can both move on. You're going to have to do it eventually, and it's much easier to yank the Band-Aid off than to stop midway because it hurts and stick it back down, only to try again later.

avoiding temptation

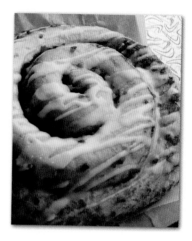

I love that saying "Nothing tastes as good as healthy feels," and I try to keep that in mind any time I feel weak.

Yesterday I was walking around IKEA and could smell the cinnamon buns. Cinnamon buns were my ultimate food in my pre–plant-based days. I loved nothing more. IKEA knew I was weak. They seemed to have cinnamon buns everywhere, and finally, I had to look at the ingredients. Could it be? Were the stars aligning?

The very last ingredient was milk. It was vegan except for that. Not plant-based— it was full of oil, processed flour, and things I couldn't easily pronounce—but, oh, if I got one without icing, it would at least be vegan! And they smelled so good! And I'd had a hard day, which had followed an already excruciating week! I'd be forgiven, right?

Then I snapped out of it. Eating that cinnamon bun wasn't going to be nearly as delicious as I remembered it to be. (I know this because I hear my clients tell me all the time, "It wasn't worth it!" and "It didn't taste as good as I remembered!" and "It was so greasy/sugary/etc.") I also knew I wouldn't feel my best and probably in thirty minutes I'd have to find a bathroom—stat! So I walked right past the cinnamon bun and decided I just liked the smell.

Now, a day later, I'm so glad I didn't eat one.

I keep strong, even in temptation, because I remember that nothing will ever taste as good as healthy feels and that there are plenty of healthy foods that I love (dehydrated mango should be illegal, it's so delicious).

I also try to remember what my old life was like (before I was thriving on plants) and how there is no amount of comfort at the bottom of a Ben & Jerry's ice cream pint that will make me feel the way plants do. I cling to that.

 When you fall down, get back up, dust yourself off, and try again. Let this motivate you to do better next time. Make the next meal a plant-based one.

And what if you goof? Follow Johnny Cash's advice: "You build on failure. You use it as a stepping stone. Close the door on the past. You don't try to forget the mistakes, but you don't dwell on it. You don't let it have any of your energy, or any of your time, or any of your space."[7]

being "selfish"

It's okay to be selfish. This is about you, not them. This is *your* health and *your* life. Your job is to take care of *you*. I'll say it again: Nothing tastes as good as healthy feels. And nothing feels as good as being true to yourself and taking care of yourself.

Remind yourself that you're no good to anyone if you're sick or not around. Put yourself first so you can be the mother/father, son/daughter, sister/brother, friend, spouse, or partner you want to be.

We also must think for ourselves and do right by ourselves because we are the ones who must live with ourselves and with the consequences of our choices.

mixed households

This question bubbles up often in my inbox—if the whole family isn't plant-based, how do you make it work? I can answer that in one word:

Compromise.

When I was a vegetarian and my husband wasn't, we agreed the house would be vegetarian, meaning he could eat whatever he wanted outside of the home (i.e., at work, at restaurants), but at home, all our meals would be vegetarian. When I went completely plant-based about a year later, my husband was fine

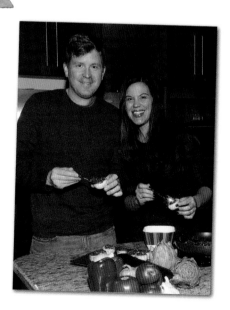

with removing eggs from our home (he wasn't much of a fan to begin with). He also used milk so infrequently that he didn't mind using soy or almond milk instead, especially when we realized that neither of us could completely use our respective "milk" before expiration. But the cheese? That wasn't going anywhere. He still wanted his cheese—along with the freedom to eat whatever he wanted outside of the home.

That was our compromise and it worked well for us. Eventually, and much to my delight, my husband went vegetarian, and then finally plant-based a few months later. Every family and situation is different, and I respect that what worked for us might not be the best solution for your household. So I asked the Herbies on Facebook that live in a mixed-diet household for advice on making it work.

Here are some of their responses:

"I'm veg, he's not. We agree on the side dishes, [then] I cook my main dish and he cooks his. We time our cooking so we can eat together."

—JULIE W.

"I'm a single mom so [the kids] have no choice. They eat what I make when we are home. I let them choose what they want when we go out."

—HEATHER S.

"Some meals are all vegan. Some meals, my husband adds meat. But I will never tell him that he cannot cook what he wants to eat in the home that we built together. The first thirty-plus years we were together, I was a meat eater too, it's not like this was a 'pre-existing condition' that he was aware of."

—SUE B.

"I have a family of five: one plant-based, one vegetarian, and three meat eaters. I cook two to three different dinners every night."

—BREN H.

"We kinda do a 50/50. Sometimes I'll cook a few vegan things I know they will eat and other times my wife makes stuff for them and I do my own thing."

—RUSS I.

"I won't buy meat. If they want it, they have to buy and prepare it."

—ROSE D.

"I am vegan and my husband is mostly paleo. He cooks all his meats on Sundays and adds them to the vegan meals I prepare throughout the week. It blends flawlessly."

—JULES B.

"I'm the only vegan in a household of eight. I knew it was going to be difficult so I took it upon myself to just cook for everyone. Who's gonna pass up an already-made meal?"

—CHRISTINE A.

"Only Herbie in a house of five people. I get one shelf in the fridge, one in the freezer, two shelves in the pantry...and I keep separate pots and pans."

—GINA C.

"I fix dinner. If the hubby and kids don't like it, they can eat it or be hungry."

—LISA C.

"I (the vegan) do all the cooking. Ninety percent of what I make can easily have meat or dairy added to it. So, it's up to him to prepare that."

—NIC T.

combatting anecdotal evidence

"My grandfather ate bacon every single day and he lived to be ninety-nine!"

You're bound to hear stories like this one—if you haven't already. It'll be the storyteller's basis for why they should disregard anything you say about why you're eating healthfully or why they should eat more plant-based foods.

I won't argue that these stories are untrue; instead, I will say that history is full of people who beat and cheat the odds. And most of us aren't as lucky.

Recently, someone said to me, "If dairy is so bad, then why is my grandma still alive at ninety-two?" I replied, "It could be any number of factors, but just because *one* person beat the odds doesn't make it true for all. I know a smoker who is ninety. Does that make cigarettes less harmful?" The asker paused and said, "Oh, I'd never thought about it that way before."

So, *one* person who ate butter and bacon (or smoked like a chimney) lived to be ninety-four. What about the hundreds and thousands of people who ate that way—or who smoked only socially—and didn't live to be fifty-four, or forty-four? If a hundred people ran across a busy highway and the only person who survived without getting hit was wearing red pants, would we all go buy red pants?

Skeptics love an anomaly. As Dr. John McDougall says, "People love to hear good news about their bad habits."[8]

This is how I combat anecdotal evidence: I explain that we all have different jars—they're different sizes and shapes, but none of us know what our jar looks like. Every time we eat animal products, a marble goes into that jar. How fast we fill it up depends on how often we eat animal products and

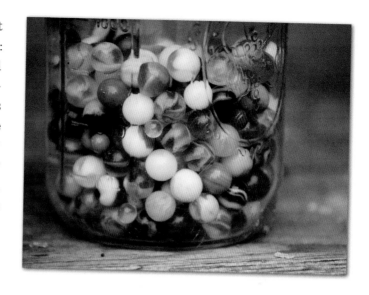

the size of our jar. But no jar is limitless. You will fill it up eventually and when you do, that's when a health crisis hits: cancer, stroke, heart disease, obesity, diabetes, and so forth.

I can't tell you what size jar you have or how fast you'll fill it up. I can only tell you that you will fill it up by eating animal products, and the only way not to

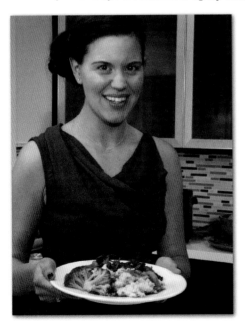

fill it up, the only way to prevent marbles from going *in* the jar, is to eat plant foods.

Scientific research even suggests that we can take marbles back *out* of the jar (so to speak) once we commit to a plant-based diet.

The reality for one person (the one who eats bacon and butter every day and lives to be ninety-nine) isn't the reality for most of us, but all of us can give ourselves the best shot. Science has proven that we can help prevent and reverse nearly all medical emergencies and sickness by simply eating plants. That is the reality for all of us and that's the reality I'm most interested in.

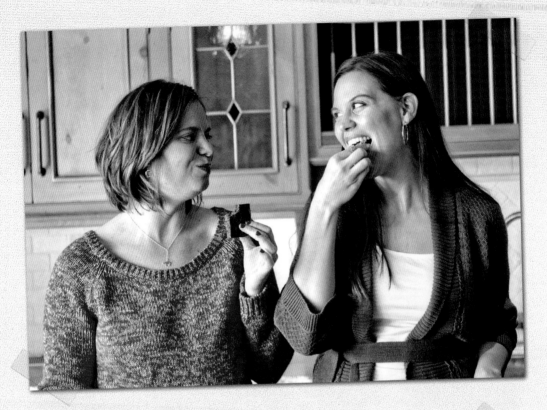

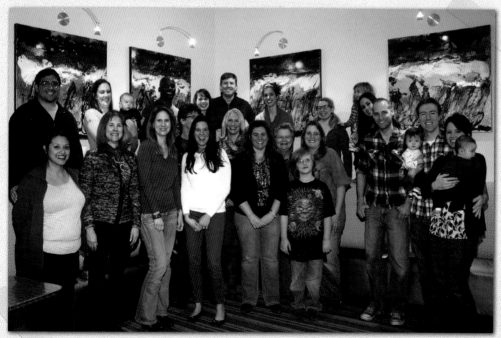

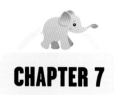

CHAPTER 7

getting family and friends on board

(lead by example)

"Our chief want is someone who will inspire us to be what we know we could be."

—RALPH WALDO EMERSON—

When I first adopted a plant-based diet, I tried to push it on my family and friends, with little success. I preached, I begged, I sent gross pictures from slaughterhouses and cringe-worthy undercover videos by PETA on YouTube. And I had zero converts.

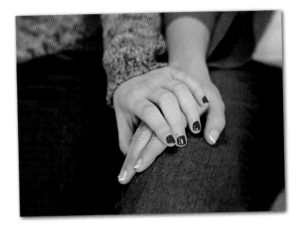

Eventually, I gave up and decided this was just going to be my own thing. Something I could keep in my pocket and feel good about—my own warm fuzzy.

Then something interesting happened: My friends and family started becoming interested. They asked me questions (with genuine interest, not teasingly) about my diet or the benefits. They hung onto my every word and soaked up the information I shared. By living and loving my lifestyle, I sparked curiosity. As I continued to thrive, lose weight, and get my glow back, they became more curious and more interested.

Within a few years, I "converted" most of my family and the majority of my friends to a plant-based or mostly plant-based diet. And those who aren't plant-based or vegetarian, I see that they are heading there.

Recently, I went out to dinner with a mixed group of friends, and one friend who I haven't known long ordered a vegan option from the menu. Another friend said, "Oh, has Lindsay gotten to you? Are you a vegan now?" He looked at me for a moment, then smiled and said, "Now that you mention it, since meeting Lindsay and Scott I am eating more vegan meals. But I ordered the vegan wrap because it's just so good." I love that! I'm always rubbing off on people.

Even friends I don't see regularly, but with whom I've stayed connected on Facebook, will send me e-mails about how they bought one of my cookbooks to support me (thanks!) and, to their surprise, they really like the food and cook from it all the time now. Or my friends will comment on my great complexion or my trim figure and say, "It's clearly working for you, so now I'm giving it a try!" I'm not exaggerating when

I say I get these e-mails every week. And all of this happened after I *stopped* preaching!

Perhaps my favorite story happened last week. My mom's best friend's daughter, Anne-Marie, was at a workshop in Tennessee. She was eating beans and rice for lunch when another attendee complimented her healthy choices. Anne-Marie explained, "A family member has been encouraging everyone to get healthy and eat more plant-based,

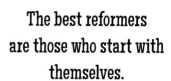

The best reformers are those who start with themselves.

—GEORGE BERNARD SHAW—

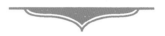

and I'm enjoying it." That's when the attendee whipped around and said, "Well then, I have to tell you about my favorite plant-based cookbook author!" It was me, and Anne-Marie beamed, saying, "Lindsay is the family member I just spoke of!" I didn't even know that Anne-Marie had been eating plant-based, or that she was following my posts on Facebook. It was an awesome moment and certainly a testament to the power of leading by example!

Living your lifestyle and thriving is the best testament and sales pitch there is.

◄ tailor your message so it's heard ►

When you want to talk to someone about the benefits of a plant-based diet, know your listener. Take a moment to consider what they are interested in and what kind of topic they might empathize with, and go in from that angle.

For example, my uncle is a hunter and would tune out anything I said about animal rights. However, he is very health conscious, so when I talk to him about eating plants, I focus on the health benefits and also the health consequences of eating meat.

On the other hand, when a friend asked me about my clear skin, and whether I had tips for what she could do to stop her acne, I kindly pointed out that dairy is a known culprit,

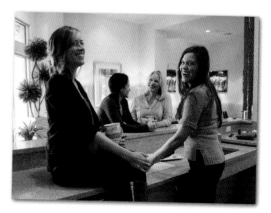

JEREMY: PLANT-PROUD DAD RAISING A PLANT-BASED FAMILY
september 2013

HH: You had a pretty rough year last year. Can you tell us about that?

To say my wife and I have had a tough year would be an understatement, but I can't imagine carrying the 79 pounds I used to carry while raising a newborn as my wife suffered and then recovered from a separated pelvis from childbirth. To top it off, I ended last year and started this year on crutches as my doctor discovered a stress fracture that I probably had since the previous summer.

HH: You've often credited the birth of your son as a big motivation for getting healthy. Can you elaborate?

I knew that I was going to be overweight in the first pictures taken of me with my son, but I also didn't want to be overweight when my son was able to make his first memories of me.

That was my motivation last January when our first and only child was born. It took until May for me to finally do something, and once I did, my motivation changed because I was feeling great and losing a ton of weight while doing something I know will give my wife and me the best chance to grow old and healthy together.

HH: What was your health like before you were plant-based, when your son was born?

Last February, right after my son was born, I found myself weighing as much as I ever knew myself to weigh: 277 pounds. My son was born with jaundice and his bilirubin was very high (high enough at one point that

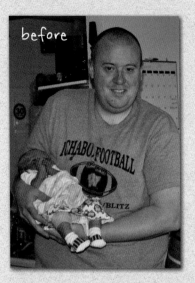

before

if it hadn't gone down after the next blood test, he would have needed a transfusion). He was released from the hospital after a couple of days, but we still had to go back every day for blood tests. We went in the morning to keep from missing too much work, and most days we would get drive-thru breakfast sandwiches. We would often go out for dinner as well to "treat" ourselves after another stressful day. The convenience of fast food and its addicting taste sure felt good as we dealt with this added stress.

HH: Your wife was also having some medical issues of her own, right?

Yes. On top of what was happening with our son, my wife was in a great deal of pain whenever she tried to walk around. Our midwife was concerned Michaela had separated her pelvis during our son's birth, so we tried basic treatment options like a pelvic binder, and she used a walker to get around. After six months of continued pain, an orthopedic doctor finally gave Michaela an X-ray and found that the gap in her pelvis was large enough that she needed surgery. A month later, she received a metal plate, some screws, and a wheelchair. Thankfully, her pain is completely gone now.

HH: Wow! That's a lot to deal with! I'm glad Michaela is feeling better. Now let's get back to you. You said it took until May for you to finally do something. What happened? What pushed you to make a change?

Last April, as my son was in his third month, I remember buying a pair of shorts. I was fed up with my body size and I just wanted something that fit comfortably. The shorts were the biggest waist size I ever bought and I truly felt like I was about to just give in and accept the fact that I was going to be a big person from then on. I don't even know why. I wasn't trying to lose weight. I just had no motivation to try anything with all that was going on. The stress of it stuck with me until the following month (May 2012), when I started tracking and limiting my calories. I had the mind-set that I could still eat whatever I wanted, just less of it. Like any strict diet you stick to for a few weeks, I lost a lot of weight.

About three weeks into this diet, Michaela and I watched *Forks Over Knives* and immediately adopted a plant-based diet that day. Since watching it, we haven't had any meat, dairy, or eggs. Also, our salt, oil, white sugar, and processed food intake is severely limited.

HH: Wow! Same day! Incredible! What was it about the documentary that was so convincing?

The warm and caring advice given in the movie by Drs. Esselstyn and Campbell convinced us that a plant-based diet is the best possible way to give our bodies the nutrition they need to get and stay healthy, and avoid the diseases that end up killing many of us (heart disease, cancer, and diabetes). The science presented in the movie and the success stories featured were enough to convince us. The higher your consumption of animal protein from meat and dairy, the higher your chances of getting the diseases I listed above and many others. Tons of studies show this, and many people think that moderation is okay. My wife and I have decided to eliminate those foods instead.

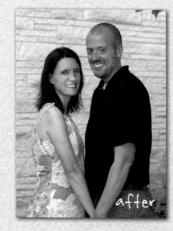

after

HH: You were "dieting" before, but did going plant-based change your approach to weight loss?

I realized that just counting and limiting calories wasn't really doing my body any good, especially if I was still eating bad food. A body doesn't really crave calories and macronutrients like protein, carbs, or fats. It really wants nutrients, and the most nutrient-rich foods are plants, which can give you all the nutrients you need. There's no need to watch carbs or proteins.

HH: What has surprised you most about the plant-based lifestyle?

I have learned since I made this change, while looking at nearly every study and article released on diet and disease prevention, that the often less talked-about group, vegans, had the lowest chances of getting serious diseases. The media doesn't want to scare off readers or viewers by telling them to give up their pizza or yogurt. Instead, they will focus on the study that says subbing 300 calories of red meat a day for 300 calories of oil will give you a lower chance of heart disease, and viewers will think they should eat oil at every meal. Sure, olive oil may be healthier than a steak, but what the stories don't look at are the numbers on the people who don't eat any animal products or oil at all. That alone has convinced me to totally cut out meat, dairy, and artificially added oil.

HH: Now the burning question: Did you keep losing weight after switching to a plant-based diet?

The weight loss has been amazing, and even after the first few months of rapid loss, I'm still losing about a pound a week eating all I want as long as it's plant-based! Resources like Happy Herbivore are really helpful in giving me new ideas and showing me that almost any basic meal can be turned into a plant-based feast! It

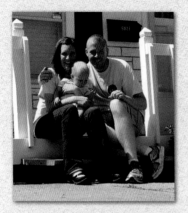

didn't take long to lose the cravings everyone imagines they would have if they went vegan. Pizza with gooey cheese was the hardest for both of us, but now I find the sight of it disgusting, and my wife is motivated by the fact that she doesn't get migraines anymore from dairy—that helps keep us away from ice cream!

HH: Who does the cooking, you or your lovely wife?

I have always done most of the cooking in the family. I love it and it can be a stress reliever for me, but I certainly find it challenging to feed all three of us, especially since my son needs more fats than we do. He gets flaxseed in his oatmeal every morning, and half an avocado every day or so. The little guy has actually eaten a whole avocado in one sitting and then went on to eat what we were having! There are days when he eats more than I do!

HH: While you're both plant-based, you and Michaela have different motivations for adopting the plant-based lifestyle. Can you tell us a little more about that?

We both jumped into this as relatively healthy individuals, so we weren't trying to lower cholesterol, blood pressure, or get off medications. I know now, though, that if I hadn't done anything, the weight could have kept going up, and we could both be on our way to the chronic diseases that so many people start to get as they grow older. Diet can cause those problems, and diet can fix them.

I went plant-based to lose weight. Michaela wants to avoid the diabetes that killed her father and uncle. We both did it to get and stay as healthy as possible.

HH: Other than your weight loss, have you or Michaela experienced any other benefits?

My cholesterol was 133 at last check. My wife hasn't had a test since giving birth, and pregnancy can skew the numbers. She was below 150 the last time she remembers.

I weigh 198 (down 79 pounds) and I now actually weigh less than what my driver's license says I weigh!

My body fat went from 39 percent in September 2011 to 24 percent when I checked it a couple months ago. The body fat scale showed that most of my weight loss has been pure fat, so I know I'm doing something right!

My wife is below her pre-pregnancy weight and hopes regrowing her muscles will help her gain some weight back.

I went from size 44 pants to 36 and an extra-large shirt to a large!

I can feel bones and muscles on my body I forgot I had, and we can get our arms around each other when we hug now.

I do sit-ups, push-ups on my knees, and other leg and arm exercises that keep me off my bad foot, and I can feel changes to my core as I do these. My hope is that by the time we're both fully recovered, we'll be well on our way to getting in the best shape of our lives, and our son will be right there with us!

UPDATE (summer 2014):

The weight I lost in the first year has stayed off completely, and I must still be doing something right, because people tell me I look like I've lost weight. I know my body fat percentage has gone down, so that must be it. My wife, son, and I still love eating plant-based foods. Our son is just over two years old and thriving. Fresh fruit is his favorite, but he also loves rice, beans, whole wheat pasta, and sauce. I enjoy packing his lunch every day for day care and finding healthy varieties without giving in to the simple, processed options.

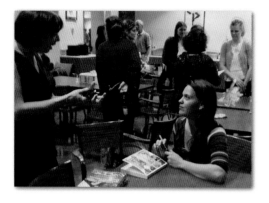

offered to send her a few studies, and suggested she go dairy-free for two weeks "just to see." When her skin cleared, she stayed off the dairy! A little while later I noticed she'd cut out all meats except fish, all on her own.

Do engage in casual, nonjudgmental conversations so you can plant a seed. Be a happy, smiling, positive, and gentle influence. Tread softly. *Don't* preach or push. Realize that you could be the person who changes their life.

Also keep in mind that the plant-based lifestyle might sound totally alien and strange to someone else. While veganism and plant-based diets are becoming more mainstream and more widely understood, they are still shockingly foreign to many people. Give your listener some time to wrap their head around the information.

I find a little bit of love goes a long way. Be upbeat and encouraging, not pushy. When friends or family try your delicious plant-based creations, thank them.

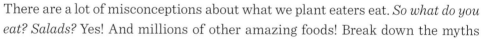

feed them (the ultimate persuasion)

There are a lot of misconceptions about what we plant eaters eat. *So what do you eat? Salads?* Yes! And millions of other amazing foods! Break down the myths and stereotypes. Show your friends and family how delicious and interesting plant-based foods are. (By the way, no one turns down muffins or desserts!) Another great idea (this one comes from my fans) is posting pictures of what you're eating and making on Facebook, Twitter, Instagram, and other social media. (To find my recipes, use the hashtag #happyherbivore or follow me

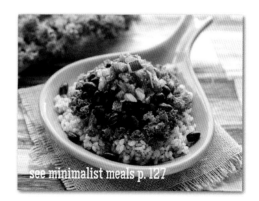

see minimalist meals p. 127

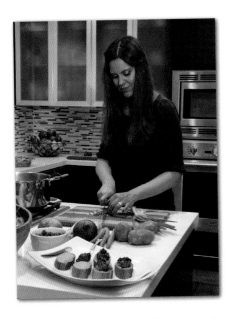

at @happyherbivore.) Show them you eat delicious, drool-worthy meals. You can keep it neutral by saying, "Dinner tonight" or "My lunch! Loved it!"

Lastly, have a movie night. Invite your friends or family over, make some plant-based snacks, and watch *Forks Over Knives, King Corn, Vegucated,* or another plant-proud documentary together. Many of these films are free on Hulu or Netflix or can be rented or purchased on Amazon.

In the end, however, the decision must be theirs. I love that saying "You can lead a horse to water but you can't make him drink." Goodness knows I've tried—especially with my parents. First trying to get them to quit smoking (which they did, eventually) and then getting them on board with a plant-based diet.

Unfortunately, it took my father having a heart attack for the plant-based diet to happen. But now that my parents are plant-based, they love it and are thriving.

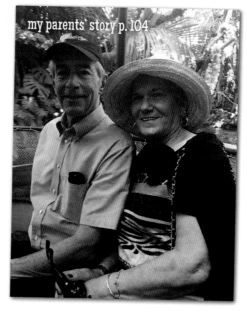

my parents' story p. 104

I wish it didn't take traumatic health events for people to make a change, but that's often what happens. (I also find going for lab work, and seeing where you stand, is often a powerful motivator. That's another approach you can take with a loved one—ask them to get their labs done.)

To summarize, keep being you. Keep leading by example. You will encourage change. It's wonderful that you care, but don't let your caring also make you angry—you'll only frustrate yourself and the person you're trying to help. As they say, you catch more flies with honey (or agave nectar) than with vinegar!

HOSTING POTLUCKS AND PARTIES

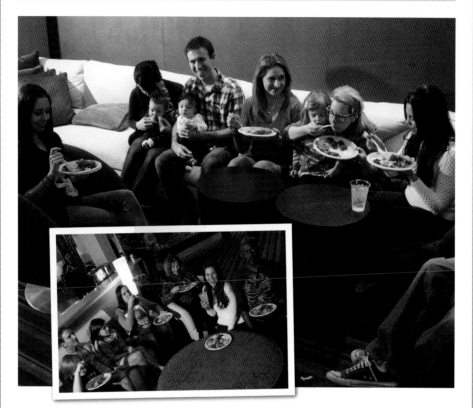

L ike tailoring your message when speaking about your lifestyle, when you're hosting, it helps to know the preferences of those you're serving. For example, I know my husband's boss loves Mexican food, so I always serve Mexican when he comes over for dinner.

If you don't know what your guests like, that's okay. The key, especially when feeding skeptical omnivores, is to serve foods that have some familiarity and "normal" ingredients they eat already—no fake meats or tofu. Go for cuisines like Mexican, Thai, or Italian that lend well to being vegetarian. (Everyone loves pasta!) Basically, don't be a "super vegan" unless you're feeding vegans or your friends are adventurous. Lastly, if you're going to a potluck or taking something in to your coworkers, take a cake, cupcakes, or muffins. No one turns down dessert!

KIM: GETTING THE FAMILY PLANT-BASED
august 2012

HH: How did you hear about a plant-based diet?

An athletic friend of mine switched to a plant-based diet and was posting her experiences on Facebook. I honestly thought, "She's lost her mind, that's extreme!" But it happened at a time when a family member of mine was quite sick from cancer, and I was thinking about how extreme the treatments are for cancer, heart disease, et cetera. (I later watched this same message in the movie *Forks Over Knives*.)

Until then, I had a fatalistic view about my risk for disease, and thought that I had no control over my chances of getting one. I felt that regardless of my exercise and a fairly good diet, genetics determined my future, instead of me taking total responsibility for what I can control. I work in a busy ER as a social worker, and I know that many things are out of our control in life. But at that moment, as I was thinking about my "extreme" vegan friend, my sick aunt was undergoing extreme cancer treatments.

One night, I was reaching into the fridge to grab a block of cheese to snack on before bed. I said to myself, "The *only* thing that I can control in this moment is what I put in my mouth to eat." I still may have a heart

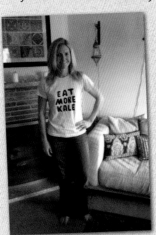

attack or get cancer, but at least I know that I tried to make a difference with my nutritional choices. I didn't eat the cheese and started to research a plant-based diet. I read *The China Study*, *Veganism for Dummies*, and a few other books, and made the switch in January 2011.

HH: You've been able to get your family on board with eating plant-based—tell us about that.

I've found that by posting photos of my food and writing little tidbits (it's usually "This Happy Herbivore cookbook has such easy recipes!"), my loved ones become interested, and then also do their own research, and they have started to change their own habits. It brings me so much joy to see my family members, from my thirty-year-old cousin (with a busy family and day-care business) to my sixty-year-old aunt—and especially my nineteen-year-old niece—start to adopt a plant-based diet.

HH: Why did you take the social media approach?

I find most people just bombard their loved ones with information. I wanted to be more than the stereotype of the weirdo San Franciscan cousin/daughter/sister/friend/niece/coworker that was taking up veganism.

There is science, research, good health, and medicine behind eating plant-based. But growing up in small-town Iowa, and living in a generally meat-centric country, ours can be a tough crowd in which to share my plant-based food experience. Food and health is such a delicate subject, at times more delicate than discussions about religion or money. I decided to post photos of the food that I make on my Facebook page, thinking that others may become interested. Instead of talking about plant-based eating, and wanting to avoid the stereotypes, I felt that photos of food were less intrusive.

At first, friends and family were mildly interested in an ingredient or food they've never had or heard of before. The food also tasted good, and that was obvious by the photos. Friends and family started to ask for recipes, the names of Lindsay's cookbooks, and started sharing. I celebrate and say "woo-hoo!" every time someone asks me about plant-based eating, because I believe it's a positive way to eat and feel good. Who doesn't want the ones we love to feel their best?

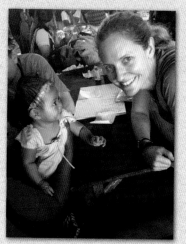

HH: Have you noticed any benefits or positive changes since making the switch?

I was physically fit to start with, but I still had health conditions that I had become used to. My cholesterol has been high since age thirteen and I've had hypothyroidism since age twenty-one. My cholesterol has improved, with my (already good) HDL jumping 14 points into the 80s. My thyroid function has improved after fourteen years of hypothyroidism, and it's become more active. Since making the switch, I've lost a few pounds and become leaner, but stayed just as strong by lifting weights and participating in athletics. I was seen by a nutritionist in December 2011 who wrote "Gorgeous!" on my analysis numbers. I get plenty of protein for my weight and activity level, as well as calcium, and all of the necessary vitamins. I'm almost

afraid to write this, but my asthma has disappeared, which I believe is linked to my acid reflux going away or not eating dairy.

Even though I was fit and at a healthy weight to start, I didn't realize the little wrong things that were adding up until they all had gone away. My mental and spiritual health have also changed for the better. You don't realize when you are eating meat and dairy what your mind and spirit can feel like by not eating animals. Eating plant-based brings a certain peace to your spirit and soul. I'm much calmer. My emotions are not as extreme as before, but I feel much more aware of my body and the world around me. I appreciate and respect all forms of life much more. This has been a big, positive change and something a lot of vegans don't discuss for fear of sounding weird!

HH: Have your family members experienced any positive benefits?

My Aunt Kathy has lost 20 pounds in the past two months and feels much better eating mostly plant-based. My Aunt Jan

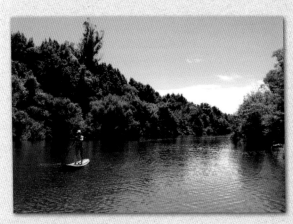

has lost 22 pounds in the past seven months and improved her other health "numbers" by eating more whole grains and more plant-based foods, and she and I both share the same love for quinoa. My cousin Brandy, in her very busy life, sets aside time to cook plant-based meals for her husband and three children. Her husband and young children are all open-minded and supportive and love Lindsay's recipe for Red Lentil Dal (*The Happy Herbivore Cookbook*, p. 73), and they've never had Indian food prior to this! I also just recently started using the meal plans and I can't believe how long I waited! I'm a planner at heart, so a whole week's worth of meals planned out and a shopping list, along with the recipes, was like an organized planner's dream come true. I find myself looking forward to a particular meal and being surprised with new recipes throughout the week. I cook most of the meals in one day, go on one shopping trip in the week, and have no stress during the week figuring out what to eat!

Posting photos of what I am eating has been the most helpful tool in my family and friends becoming interested in plant-based eating. I even post photos of four pots simmering on the stove when I'm making my meals, or of my meal at my desk at work. It shows that the meal plans and plant-based foods can be straightforward and work into a busy and active life well.

HH: Any additional comments or advice for others?

We live in one of the most fortunate times and in one of the most abundant countries on Earth. There is no reason that a person has to settle for not feeling fantastic. We have everything at our fingertips, from information about nutrition, to choice, to being able to buy almost any food at our local stores, farmers' markets, or online. I encourage others to try plant-based eating for a week, a month, or longer. Take it on as a learning experience, and you will eat a larger variety of foods than you ever thought possible.

UPDATE (summer 2014):

I continue to teach boxing, work as a social worker, respond to humanitarian disasters (as a disaster mental health specialist), and paddle-board. I am excited to be starting a new boxing program,

which is a non-contact boxing program for people with Parkinson's disease (called Rock Steady Boxing). More friends have become more plant-based because of my sharing on social media, specifically my friend Israel, who is a muscular, early-fifties, amateur boxer who just competed in the Golden Gloves tournament, and told me last week that he is staying plant-based even though his heavy training is over. I've also been dating my fantastic boyfriend, Mark (we will likely tie the knot in the future!), and our first date was at a local vegan restaurant. He's also adopted a more plant-based diet and makes fantastic grilled veggies for me that I take to work with me on Mondays and that everyone raves about (the smell and taste!).

I have dealt with severe depression in the past two years but have been healthy and in remission from the depression in the past six months. I have reexamined things along the way with my health and have not remained 100 percent vegan but still consume 99 percent plant-based foods. Lindsay's sharing of her own health problems, and especially about not being perfect, has been an inspiration to find what works for me. It also helped when I was deployed to the Philippines in November and December 2013 for disaster response to be open to eating whatever is available in a large-scale disaster, knowing that strict veganism would not help me cope with a very difficult situation where I needed to help others.

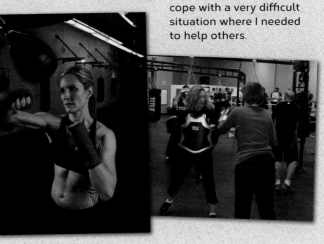

CHAPTER 8

cooking, baking, and dealing with allergies

"The cool thing is that now that people have made this evolution where cooking is cool, people are doing it on weekends, they're doing their own challenges. It's back to cooking. And it's real cooking."

—EMERIL LAGASSE—

It's time to eat! Before I was plant-based I barely knew how to boil water to make pasta, and now I'm happiest in the kitchen, cooking up culinary delights. In this chapter I'll walk you through adapting old recipes, show you the ins and outs of plant-based cooking and baking (including how to replace oil), and discuss what to do when you have allergies or need to make a substitution.

making substitutions and adaptations in recipes

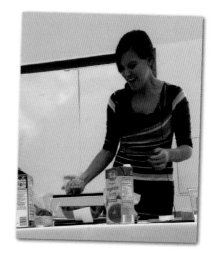

When making a substitution or an adaptation, think about what that ingredient does and ask yourself if the proposed replacement is similar in taste, consistency, color, and the like.

For example, let's say a burger recipe calls for kidney beans. You're allergic. What's a good alternative? Black beans and navy beans are similar in texture and consistency (wet, mushy) compared to the firmer, drier chickpea or black-eyed pea. Now let's think color. Black beans would probably look better visually (we eat with our eyes) than white beans in a burger, but without making a final decision, let's also ponder taste.

Would the flavors and seasonings in the recipe mesh well with the black beans? With white beans? For a curry flavor, for example, white beans would be better. For a more neutral, spicy, or Mexican flavor, black beans would be better. Think about the flavors that are usually associated with each bean to decide.

PLANT-BASED REPLACEMENTS »

Here are some quick and easy stand-ins that work in most recipes. Of course you can try to use imitation meats and faux cheeses (homemade or commercially made; see "Commercial Substitutes" in chapter four for options) for meat and cheese, but mushrooms, beans, nuts, and veggies do a great job, too!

ANIMAL INGREDIENT	PLANT-BASED CONVERSION
CHICKEN	chickpeas, white mushrooms
GROUND BEEF	black beans, bulgur, quinoa, textured vegetable protein
EGGS (SCRAMBLES, OMELET, QUICHE, ETC.)	tofu
EGGS (BAKING)	See "Replacing Eggs" (p. 200)
MILK	soy milk, almond milk, etc.
BUTTER (COOKING)	vegetable broth or water
BUTTER (BAKING)	See "Replacing Fat" (p. 201)
BUTTERMILK	soy milk combined with lemon juice or apple cider vinegar (1 cup to 1 teaspoon ratio)
BEEF STRIPS OR STEAK	portobello mushrooms
HAM	maple syrup plus smoked paprika to taste
FISH	kelp, seaweed
SEAFOOD	seaweed, Old Bay seasoning
BACON	liquid smoke to taste
CREAM	silken tofu, coconut milk, soy milk
CHEESE	miso; nutritional yeast to taste can help add flavor; and cashew cream, too
MAYO	Vegan Mayo (p. 239) or commercial substitutes
HONEY (FOR VEGANS)	agave, apple syrup, maple syrup
MEAT (GENERALLY)	seitan, tempeh, tofu
BEEF OR CHICKEN STOCK	Happy Herbivore No-Beef Broth and No- Chicken Broth (p. 238)
SOUR CREAM	plain vegan yogurt (p. 242, or commercially sold vegan sour cream such as Tofutti)
GELATIN	agar agar

allergies and allergy-free cooking

Three of the most common food allergens (dairy, seafood, and eggs) are totally avoided with a plant-based diet. Tree nuts/peanuts, wheat/gluten, and soy are plant-based foods, but they, too, and any other plant-food allergy (e.g., mango, or in my case, broccoli), can be worked around fairly easily.

I find that, when dealing with allergies, the most important thing you can do is switch your mind-set to "abundance," not "deprivation." (Think of all the food options you *can* have, rather than focus on what's off limits.)

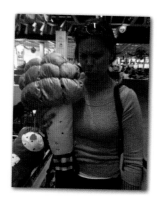

Second, don't seek out "heartbreak" recipes. I'm allergic to broccoli so I don't go looking for broccoli soups or casseroles with broccoli, because I just know I'll be disappointed. If you're allergic to beans, search for mushroom burgers or lentil burgers—skip the heartbreak of looking at a bunch of bean burger recipes you'd have to adapt. There are plenty of allergy-friendly choices out there!

soy alternatives

I find people assume if you are vegan or vegetarian you have to eat soy (tofu, soy milk), which is not true. You can be completely plant-based and never eat soy (I rarely do).

You can usually omit edamame (soybeans) in any recipe that calls for it, since it's usually just tossed in. Coconut aminos are a terrific substitute for soy sauce, shoyu, and tamari; and chickpea miso (available at most health food stores) is a soy-free miso. Quinoa and couscous are also great stand-ins for textured vegetable protein (TVP), and are more wholesome options, too!

Commercial substitutes: Instead of soy milk, buy rice milk, oat milk, hemp milk, almond milk, or any other plant-based, nondairy milk. (You can also find coconut-, rice-, and almond-based yogurts, ice creams, and other vegan dairy substitutes.) Smiling Hara Tempeh and the Hearty Vegan both make soy-free tempehs made from beans. Living Harvest also makes a hemp-based soy-free tofu, and you can find recipes online for making soy-free tofu from chickpea (garbanzo bean) flour.

Recipe substitutions: If the recipe calls for silken (soft) tofu, you can try using a vegan yogurt. If firm or extra-firm tofu is called for, you can try using white beans or potatoes.

My 7-Day Meal Plans (http://www.getmealplans.com) are always soy-free if you need more ideas.

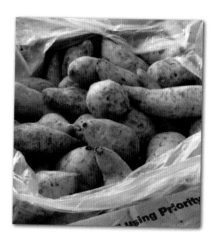

nut alternatives

Nuts and seeds are easily avoidable on a plant-based diet. I rarely use either in my recipes or cookbooks. Sunflower seeds and sunflower seed butter, as well as soy-nut–based butters, are a great replacement for peanut butters and tree nut butters should you need one. In most recipes, nuts can be omitted without too much compromise. For example, a banana-walnut bread will still be delicious without the walnuts. I also find that beans, particularly white beans, can stand in for nuts like pine nuts or walnuts in most savory recipes.

My 7-Day Meal Plans (http://www.getmealplans.com) are always nut-free if you need more ideas.

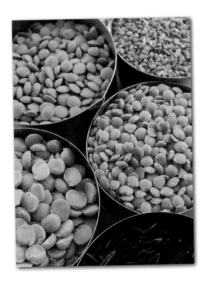

legume (beans and lentils) alternatives

In many recipes you can leave out the legumes without much trouble. For example, if a vegetable stew calls for white beans, you can omit the beans without ruining the stew.

If you're allergic to beans but not lentils (or vice versa) try using the other. You can also get creative with vegetable combinations. Let's say you found a great recipe for black bean enchiladas but you're allergic to beans. Why not make kale and sweet potato enchiladas instead? Or lentil enchiladas? (Wondering where you'll get your protein? *See "The Protein Myth" in chapter one.*)

wheat and gluten alternatives

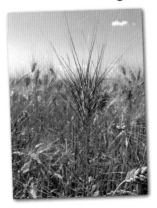

These days, you can walk into almost any grocery store and find gluten-free pasta on the shelf. Most supermarkets have a gluten-free section or gluten-free goods on the shelf next to wheat products. Even more options exist in health food stores or online.

Gluten-free grains like brown rice and quinoa are a great replacement for barley, farro, couscous, and other grains that contain wheat or gluten. Tamari is a great wheat-free, gluten-free alternative to soy sauce and shoyu, as are coconut aminos, which are also soy-free.

If you're looking to make seitan ("wheat meat") or if a recipe calls for vital wheat gluten, you can use Orgran's gluten-free gluten substitute, available online and at some health food stores. There's also a recipe for homemade gluten-free gluten (seitan) on HappyHerbivore.com.

My 7-Day Meal Plans (http://www.getmealplans.com) are always gluten-free if you need more ideas.

See "Gluten-Free Baking" later in this chapter for more information.

corn alternatives

Corn kernels can usually be left out of a recipe without causing a problem. Instead of cornstarch, use arrowroot or potato starch, available at some supermarkets and most health food stores. Instead of a corn tortilla, try using a flour tortilla.

In recipes calling for a tiny bit of cornmeal, you can usually use almond meal or a wheat-based flour like white whole-wheat flour or all-purpose flour. If a lot of cornmeal is called for, say, to make cornbread, you could try using millet or a ground millet flour.

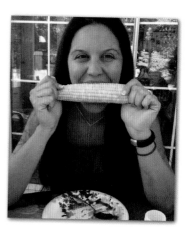

alternatives for other foods

Except for mushrooms and miso (sorry—no substitutes exist for those items!), most ingredients have a plant-based cousin that can stand in for them.

For example, if you're allergic to mango, try using peaches. Use cauliflower instead of potatoes, butternut squash or carrots instead of sweet potatoes, and so on. Try doing a web search of "substitute for [food name]" and be dazzled by your options. One of my frequent, go-to resources is The Cook's Thesaurus online (foodsubs.com). All-Recipes.com also has a helpful substitutions table.

plant-based baking

If you're looking to adapt an old family recipe to be vegan (but not necessarily plant-based or healthier), it's pretty easy. Flour is vegan and sugar is usually fine.[i] Butter can be replaced with vegan margarine (a popular brand is Earth Balance), but some margarines may contain dairy or animal products, so check the label. Eggs can also be substituted out fairly easily, too (more on that soon).

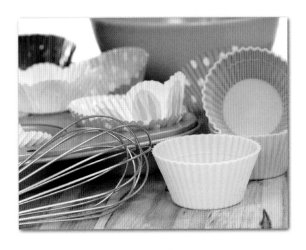

Adapting a recipe to be plant-based and healthy (or at least, healthier) and oil-free is where it gets a little tricky, but it's still possible.

If you're a novice baker I recommend trying a recipe that's already vegan or plant-based before adapting a recipe beyond substituting butter and eggs. For example, if you're hungry for Mom's blueberry muffins, try making the blueberry muffins in *Happy Herbivore Light & Lean* first. Once you're more comfortable with

---

i. Since white sugar can be processed through bone char, strict vegans may not use it. Certified vegan white sugar is available at health food stores.

baking, start adapting old recipes. I also find that studying already vegan recipes as a reference can be very helpful.

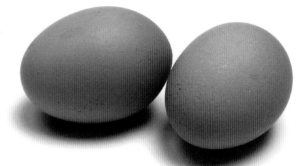

replacing eggs

To replace one egg, use:

¼ CUP APPLESAUCE	Add with wet ingredients. Avoid using more than 1 cup total applesauce in a recipe. Applesauce works best in breads, muffins, and cakes.
½ BANANA, MASHED	Cream banana with sugar or blend with liquids. The riper the banana, the sweeter it'll be and the more banana flavor you'll have.
2½ TABLESPOONS GROUND FLAXSEEDS MIXED WITH 3 TABLESPOONS WATER AND CHILLED FOR 15 MINUTES	Add as you would an egg in the original recipe. Note that flax has an earthy flavor, which is not always complementary.
1 TABLESPOON GROUND CHIA SEEDS WHISKED WITH 3 TABLESPOONS WATER	Let it sit for ten minutes, or until it develops into a goop. Add as you would an egg in the original recipe. You can find chia seeds at most supermarkets and all health food stores.
¼ CUP (2 OUNCES) SILKEN TOFU OR VEGAN YOGURT	Blend with liquids. Warning: Tofu and yogurt can be very heavy, so don't use in "fluffy" or delicate recipes like pancakes, or where multiple eggs must be replaced.

Commercial substitutes: Ener-G-Egg Replacer is sold at most health food stores and online. Orgran also makes a No Egg egg replacer, though it's harder to find. "The Vegg" is another brand that offers both a completely plant-based egg yolk substitute and a baking mix. These substitutes can be helpful when you're new to baking and feeling overwhelmed by substitutions, but overall I find them unnecessary and a bit pricey. Some people also complain they leave a chalky taste (see online reviews for the products).

To replace one egg white: Use 1 tablespoon agar agar powder (sold at health food stores and Asian supermarkets) dissolved into 1 tablespoon water. Whip it, chill it, then whip it again.

replacing fat (butter, margarine, shortening, and oil)

SUBSTITUTE	BEST USE	WARNING	HOW TO USE
APPLESAUCE	Cakes, cupcakes, some cookies	Avoid using more than 1 cup of applesauce in any recipe	Use slightly less than the amount of fat originally called for
CANNED PURE PUMPKIN	Muffins, some cupcakes, chocolate-flavored treats, oatmeal cookies	Adds a hint of pumpkin flavor & an orange color	Use the same amount as originally called for, plus an extra splash of liquid
AVOCADO	For cookies that need a "crisp" crumble	Adds a green color & is high in fat	Replace ½ the fat called for with avocado or peanut butter, then ¼ the fat called for with applesauce or banana
PEANUT BUTTER		Adds a hint of peanut butter flavor & is high in fat	
BANANA	Cookies, biscuits, scones	The greener the banana, the better	Use in place of shortening when you need to "cut" fat in

Reducing the baking temperature to 350°F for muffins, breads, and cakes can help your fat-free goodies retain moisture. You might want to reduce it even lower for cookies and bars, since a longer, slower bake time can help make them a little firmer.

whole-wheat flours

I use white whole-wheat flour and whole-wheat pastry flour in my baking recipes instead of white flour (all-purpose flour). The most nutritious parts of flour—the wheat seed, bran, and germ—have all been removed from white flour. In fact, white flour is so devoid of nutrients after processing that the FDA requires manufacturers to artificially add some nutrition back in. (This is why it's called "enriched" flour.)

Whole-wheat flours still contain all their nutrients, making them more healthful. Regular whole-wheat flour (as opposed to white whole-wheat flour or whole-wheat pastry flour) is made from red wheat, which is why it's dark in color. Red-wheat flour is also dense and grainy, so it's great for hearty breads but not for baked goods. Regular whole-wheat flour is also much "thirstier" than all-purpose flour, so if you don't add extra liquid when adapting a recipe, you might end up with dense, brick-hard goodies. I generally don't recommend using regular whole-wheat flour in baking, especially if you are a novice baker.

White whole-wheat flour, on the other hand, is made from white wheat, a different kind of grain. White wheat is softer and lighter, making it perfect for baked goods and a nutritious alternative to all-purpose flour. Your baked goods won't be as light and fluffy as they would be with all-purpose, but they'll be much lighter and airier than if you used regular whole-wheat flour. Most supermarkets carry white whole-wheat flour. Arnold's is my favorite brand, followed by Bob's Red Mill (which makes my favorite whole-wheat pastry flour, too). Whole-wheat pastry flour, which you can find in most health food stores, is even lighter. It's made from red wheat but has a lower gluten content.

Lastly, always spoon flour from the bag lightly into a measuring cup, and then gently level off with a knife. Do not scoop the flour out of the bag with your measuring cup, "pack" the flour down, or "tap" the measuring cup. This will cause you to have too much flour, which will make your baked goods dense. For more information and a tutorial video, see "Baking Perfection, Troubleshooting Tips" on HappyHerbivore.com.[ii]

gluten-free baking

The easiest way to convert a recipe to be gluten-free is to use a gluten-free all-purpose flour blend such as Bob's Red Mill Gluten-Free All Purpose Flour, or another commercial brand. Unfortunately, you can't use a gluten-free flour such as chickpea flour or rice flour in a straight 1:1 ratio for all-purpose or whole-wheat flours. You need to use a binder such as xanthan gum. A blend of different gluten-free flours also works best. If you need a recipe to be wheat-free but not gluten-free, you can use spelt flour (but know

A note about paper liners:

Skip liners and use nonstick pans and silicon bakeware if you can. You can also line cookie sheets and muffin cups with parchment paper. (Some health food stores sell disposable liners made from parchment paper.) If you use traditional paper liners, they won't peel easily while the goodies are still hot. If you let it cool completely and wait a few hours, it will peel away perfectly.

that it has a "nutty" taste) or oat flour. To make oat flour, pulverize instant ("quick") or old-fashioned ("rolled") oats in your blender until you have a flour consistency.

sugar and sweeteners

I'm of the opinion that sugar is sugar. I try to use the least processed sweetener I can, but I still recognize that all sweeteners should only accent my diet and not play a large role—sweeteners are not health foods.

Pure maple syrup is the least processed of all commercially sold sweeteners, but I find the taste is not always complementary in every recipe. You also can't use a "wet" sweetener in place of a "dry" sweetener without making other changes to the recipe, and let's be honest: Maple syrup can be expensive.

---

ii. www.happyherbivore.com/2013/12/baking-perfection-troubleshoot-tips-vegan-egg-free

When I need a dry or a mild-tasting sweetener I tend to reach for raw sugar (also called turbinado sugar) or sucanat, since these sweeteners are more natural and slightly less processed than white sugar.

Brown sugar and confectioner's sugar (also called powdered sugar) are made from white sugar, but you can make brown sugar and powdered sugar from raw sugar at home. To make brown sugar, beat 1 tablespoon molasses into 1 cup raw sugar. To make powdered sugar, combine 1 cup raw sugar with 2 tablespoons cornstarch (arrowroot also works). Using a high-speed blender, pulverize it into powdered sugar. (Make sure your lid is on tight or you'll have a mess!)

Agave nectar is a more neutral-tasting liquid sweetener than maple syrup, and is sweeter tasting. Ethical vegans who abstain from honey commonly use agave nectar as a substitution. There is some controversy about agave and whether it is healthier than sugar and high-fructose corn syrup, but I still use agave nectar in a few token dishes.

Date syrup, while not the easiest to come by in a store, is very easy to make at home and is the healthiest and least processed liquid sweetener. To make date syrup, soak dates in hot water for at least ten minutes (overnight is best). Drain off the water but save it. Add dates to your blender with some of the water. With the motor running, add more date water as necessary until you have a syrup consistency. You can add cinnamon and vanilla extract if desired. Other liquid and dry sweeteners, which you can find at the health food store, include coconut sugar, maple sugar, brown rice syrup, and barley malt syrup.

cocoa

Most unsweetened cocoas are vegan—they're just cocoa. Hershey's is available at most supermarkets. I splurge and buy Ghirardelli unsweetened cocoa, which is also available at most supermarkets. Any brand of unsweetened cocoa will work in recipes calling for cocoa.

white chocolate

Vegan white chocolate isn't easy to come by in stores but you can generally find it online. Two brands to look for are King David Kosher Vegan and Oppenheimer.

chocolate chips

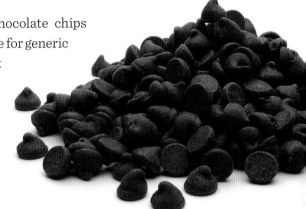

Most semisweet and unsweetened chocolate chips are vegan. (This seems particularly true for generic brands.) I like Ghirardelli semisweet chocolate chips best. If you need an allergy-free chocolate chip (soy-free, gluten-free, etc.), look for Enjoy Life chips at health food stores and online. Enjoy Life also makes mini chocolate chips.

carob

If you're looking to avoid caffeine, carob powder and carob chips (available at most health food stores) make good chocolate substitutes. The taste isn't *the same* but it's as close as you can get. Two caveats: Carob, unlike chocolate, is naturally sweet, so you may need to reduce your sweetener in a recipe if you substitute carob for chocolate or cocoa. Carob also burns more easily while cooking, so you might want to reduce your oven temp by 25°F.

milk

I find that almond milk and soy milk work best in baking. (*See "Transition Tips" in chapter four for general information on nondairy milk.*)

 If you're looking for a lower-fat coconut milk, try adding a drop or two of coconut extract to your nondairy milk of choice. You may also want to add 1 teaspoon of cornstarch to thicken it.

GINA: LOST MORE THAN 100 POUNDS BY SWITCHING FROM "VEGAN" TO PLANT-BASED

february 2013

HH: Most people who adopt a plant-based diet transition from the Standard American Diet, but you already were vegan. Tell us a little about that.

I stopped eating meat when I was thirteen, for ethical reasons. I became vegan shortly after that, at nineteen (after reading John Robbins' *Diet for a New America*). That said, I was not a healthy vegan. I gave up meat, but never really understood how to "balance" meals and make them healthy. I ended up living on "side dishes," and if I went out to eat with friends? I ate French fries, soda, pasta, and if I was "lucky," bread. So, unlike almost everyone else who goes vegan, I *gained* weight. A LOT of weight. I never felt like I was a "good" representative of the vegan lifestyle, and for many of my friends, I'm the only vegan they know. Why would anyone else want to follow in my footsteps, when I looked like I did?

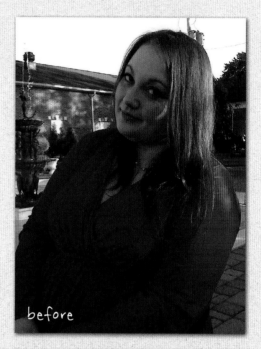

before

HH: Other than the weight, did you have any other health issues?

I had many other "issues" in regard to my health. I had lots of gastrointestinal problems, and this persistent rash on my fingers that blistered and caused them to crack and become very painful.

HH: How did you find your way to a plant-based diet?

It was only in researching this skin issue on the internet (after having gone to a dermatologist, being diagnosed with eczema, handed steroid creams, and being told there was nothing more that could be done except treat it topically) that I stumbled on a site that showed something that looked remarkably like my rash but called it "dermatitis herpetiformis."

Further, the website claimed it was a hallmark of celiac disease. *What?!?*

I couldn't possibly be allergic to wheat. *I live on wheat products. I'm vegan!*

I read the list of symptoms and had many of them. I figured I had nothing to lose by trying to give up wheat for a while, to see if anything changed. I don't think it took more than a week for the rash on my fingers to disappear. I couldn't remember a time when I didn't have it, and it was gone. That alone changed everything.

HH: How so?

I made the decision to return to college and finish my degree. As you can imagine, I became incredibly busy and often missed lunch. (I do not recommend doing that, but it happens.) I figured if breakfast was the only meal I'd have until dinner, I'd better make sure breakfast was something better than a plate of tater tots (tater tots are vegan and gluten-free!). I started Googling for recipes that were both vegan and gluten-free, and I came across Happy Herbivore.

Some of the first recipes I cooked were from the website, and they're still the ones I recommend to people who are looking to try out plant-based eating: Hippie Loaf, Quiche with Greens, even the Dirty Mashed Potatoes. Because serving sizes were something that always challenged me, I loved how Happy Herbivore spelled everything out so easily. I made the recipes, and portioned them out into containers in the fridge so my meals were set to be heated up and eaten in a hurry.

Then I bought the Happy Herbivore cookbooks and found many, many more new favorite recipes. I think I own literally every vegan cookbook on the market, and they all end up gathering dust on my bookshelf, mainly because *the recipes are incredibly complicated*. But Happy Herbivore recipes are different. They're amazing, delicious, simple, easy, fast, and healthy. My m.o. became this: Cook on Sunday, fill the refrigerator, and eat from the already portioned-out containers all week long.

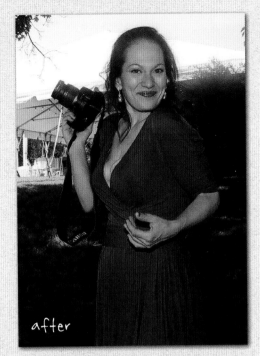

after

HH: Aww, you are too kind! So when did the weight loss start happening?

Before I even knew it, my jeans were getting looser. Then I needed a belt. Then I needed a smaller belt. I dared to step on the scale and was amazed at how much I'd lost. I gave myself a goal, and declared that when I reached it, I'd start exercising. I met the number just as last summer began and started walking every day. I felt like I'd come out of a fog. I never knew how sick I was, until I wasn't.

Somewhere in there, you launched your meal plan service, the 7-Day Meal Plans (http://www.getmealplans.com). I started buying them, even though I had the cookbooks, because these meal plans were portioned out to single or double servings. I don't have to do math anymore. You even include gluten-free alternatives for me. I don't even have to think! I just buy what's on the list, and make the meals, and I'm still losing weight. As I'm typing this, I've lost 133 pounds, and I'm only about 10 pounds from what I think is my end goal.

HH: That is incredible! Congrats! Did you ever expect your life to turn out this way?

If someone had told me even a year ago that I would be buying jeans in a *size 4*, I would have laughed—but that totally just happened. And it would never, ever have happened on my own, without you! You have honestly changed my entire way of life. I can now say I *am* a good example of a vegan. I post pictures of the meals I cook, and in fact, many of my friends are asking about what I'm doing. (I always direct them right to you!)

HH: Anything else you'd like to add?

I hope you know what a huge difference you make in the lives of others. You have literally changed my life! (And now, you have given me crêpes and anise cookies and so many other new things I cannot wait to try!) Thank you!!!

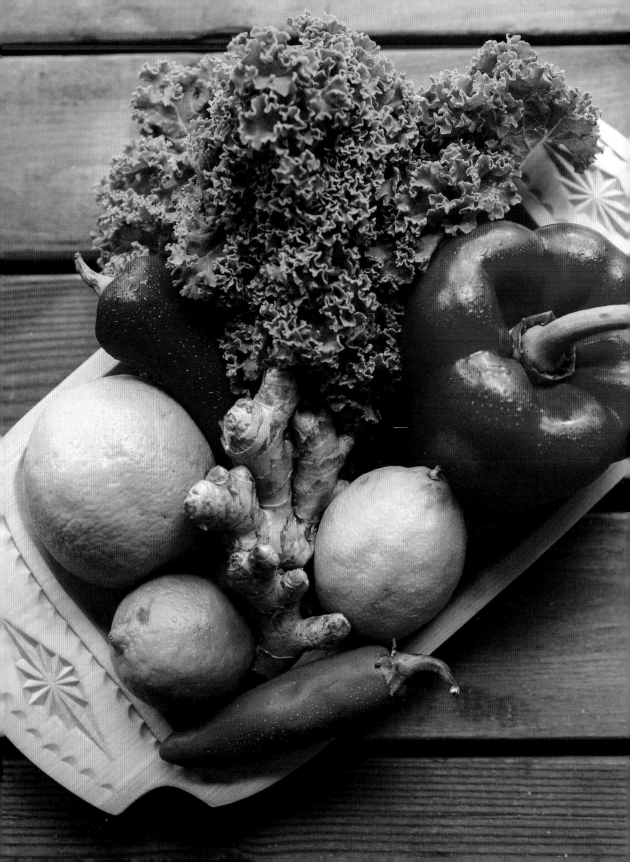

CHAPTER 9

troubleshooting:
failure to thrive

"Our greatest weakness lies in giving up.
The most certain way to succeed is always to
try just one more time."

–THOMAS A. EDISON–

Occasionally people will come to me saying they tried a vegan diet or a plant-based diet but they didn't feel well, they lacked energy, they didn't lose weight, and so forth. Basically, they "failed to thrive." They didn't experience all the amazing benefits they heard about or expected to feel on a plant-based diet. *What gives?*

First, remember that anyone who makes a change in their diet (even a positive change) will experience the symptoms of that change. Some individuals feel great immediately, others have a few rough days or even weeks while they detox—your body is flushing out the toxins and adjusting to this change. We all come to a plant-based lifestyle from a different place, so what might be a small change for one person could be a huge change for someone else. Your experience is unique to you! *(See "A Note about Cravings" in chapter six for more information on withdrawal and feeling lousy.)*

That said, there are a few factors—common culprits—that can make someone fail to thrive. I'll discuss each in turn. To quote an often repeated saying, "There is no sadder or more frequent obituary on the pages of time than, 'We have always done it this way.'"

issue: not losing weight

The number-one culprit for stalled weight loss (or weight gain) is oil and added fats. Oil can sneak into all kinds of foods you'd never expect, like condiments and breads. Eliminate all oils. Also be mindful of (and cut back on) high-fat plant foods. As Dr. John McDougall says, "The fat you eat is the fat you wear." If you're trying to lose fat, don't eat more of it. Cut back on nuts, seeds, avocado, nut butters (e.g., peanut butter or almond butter), coconut milk, chocolate, olives, and soy. Other culprits include liquid calories (alcohol, coffee, smoothies, and juices), dried fruits (use sparingly for flavor, not as a snack), fiber-broken foods (choose whole grains like rice over flours), eating out at restaurants, and convenience "vegan" foods such as imitation meats, excess salt, and sugar.

In all my years as a personal trainer and in offering a meal plan service to clients, I have found time and time again that diet is the problem *and* the solution. It matters *what* you eat far more than how much you eat (i.e., total calories).

issue: feeling tired and irritable

If you feel fatigued and irritable, first check to make sure you're eating enough calories. Big bowls of vegetables are healthy and awesome—and filling!—but can add up to barely 500 calories. This means you can easily stuff yourself while also being calorically deficient, which isn't going to leave you feeling energized or at your best.

I find that clients who were dieters or previously restricted their calories tend to fall into this trap the most. Because most plant foods are so low in calories, the total volume of food you eat in a day will go up. Personally, I love this aspect about a plant-based diet: It's really about abundance, not deprivation! But if you're accustomed to smaller portions, you can very easily eat too few calories.

Even if you haven't restricted your diet in the past, you can still undereat accidentally, and then you won't feel your best. Also make sure you're including healthy starches: cooked grains (like rice) and potatoes. (This is a common solution for my "fatigued" clients.) These should form the bulk of your diet—see my pyramid (page 36).

If you need help and guidance, check out my 7-Day Meal Plans (www.getmealplans.com); they make it so easy to do the plant-based diet right.

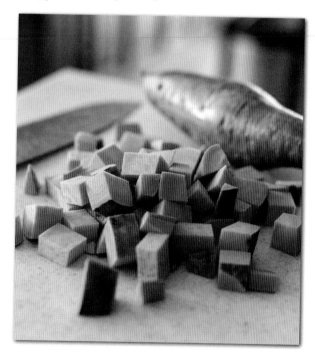

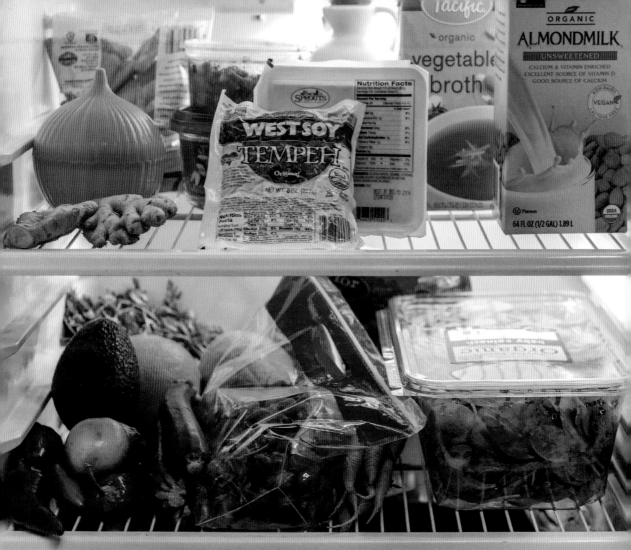
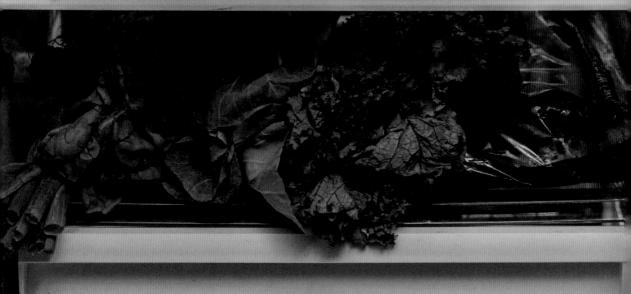

CHAPTER 10

getting started on your plant-based journey

"Every new beginning comes from
some other beginning's end."

—SENECA—

make a commitment

DON'T *GO* ON A DIET. *CHANGE* YOUR DIET.

From my own personal experience, as well as my experience working with hundreds of clients, I can attest that there has to be a serious commitment to see real, lasting results. Make a lifelong commitment to thriving. Choose yourself. Choose yourself over convenience. Choose yourself over peer pressure. Choose yourself over the ease, familiarity, and comfort of deep-rooted, bad habits. Choose to believe that you are not a helpless victim. Appreciate and understand that you can vote for health with every bite (that fork is mighty powerful!) and that this year can be your best yet!

By now, as you're nearing the end of this book you are probably well on your way (or about to be!) on your own marvelous plant-based journey. Because it *is* a journey. (More on that soon!)

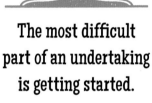

The most difficult part of an undertaking is getting started.

−UNKNOWN−

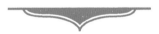

just begin

Nike got it right. Don't overthink it, *just do it*! Make the next thing you eat, whether it's a snack or a meal, a plant food. Don't wait for the perfect moment or a surge of inspiration—just do it! You don't need to get your ducks in a row. You don't need to finish eating what's in the freezer (throw it away or gift it to a friend—your health is a greater investment). You don't need to do *anything* else. You just need to start eating plants. Today is your day! With each baby step you build momentum! Fuel that healthy fire!

shopping list

See Gluten-free list for items with an *.

breads and dry goods

- [ ] brown rice
- [ ] couscous
- [ ] lentils
- [ ] quinoa
- [ ] red lentils
- [ ] yellow split peas

canned goods

- [ ] black beans
- [ ] chickpeas (garbanzo beans)
- [ ] coconut milk (lite)
- [ ] green chilies (4 oz)
- [ ] kidney beans
- [ ] pineapple (crushed, diced)
- [ ] pumpkin (pure, *not* pumpkin pie filling)
- [ ] refried beans (vegetarian)
- [ ] tomato paste
- [ ] tomato sauce
- [ ] tomatoes (diced)
- [ ] white beans (e.g., navy beans, cannellini beans, butter beans)

condiments and dressings

- [ ] apple cider vinegar
- [ ] balsamic vinaigrette (fat-free; optional)
- [ ] barbecue sauce
- [ ] Dijon mustard
- [ ] hot sauce (e.g., Cholula, Tabasco)
- [ ] hot sauce (Asian; e.g., Sriracha)
- [ ] hummus (optional)
- [ ] ketchup
- [ ] miso (yellow or white, *not* brown)
- [ ] pineapple salsa
- [ ] salsa (regular)
- [ ] soy sauce (low sodium)*
- [ ] sweet red chili sauce
- [ ] Worcestershire sauce (vegan; optional)
- [ ] yellow mustard

soy and nondairy

- [ ] nondairy milk (e.g., soy, rice, almond)
- [ ] tempeh
- [ ] tofu (firm and extra-firm)
- [ ] yogurt (vegan; plain and flavored)

fresh produce

- [ ] apples
- [ ] avocado (optional)
- [ ] bananas
- [ ] bell peppers

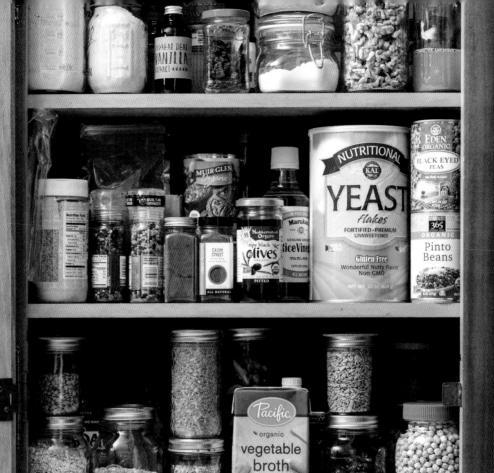
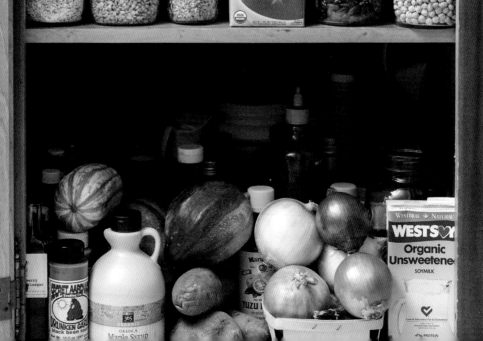

- ☐ blueberries (or frozen)
- ☐ broccoli (or frozen)
- ☐ cabbage
- ☐ carrots
- ☐ celery
- ☐ cucumber
- ☐ garlic cloves
- ☐ ginger root
- ☐ grapes
- ☐ green onions
- ☐ greens (e.g., kale, collard greens, spinach, lettuce)
- ☐ herbs (e.g., basil, cilantro, mint, oregano, thyme)
- ☐ jalapeños
- ☐ lemons
- ☐ limes
- ☐ mango
- ☐ mushrooms
- ☐ onions (red and yellow)
- ☐ oranges
- ☐ potatoes
- ☐ spaghetti squash
- ☐ strawberries (fresh or frozen)
- ☐ sweet potatoes
- ☐ tomatoes
- ☐ zucchini

freezer

- ☐ corn
- ☐ edamame

- ☐ fruit (e.g., blueberries, strawberries)
- ☐ greens (e.g., spinach)
- ☐ mixed vegetables
- ☐ peas
- ☐ pineapple chunks
- ☐ stir-fry vegetables

pantry

- ☐ almond extract
- ☐ applesauce (unsweetened)
- ☐ artichoke hearts
- ☐ black olives
- ☐ brown rice
- ☐ green olives
- ☐ Kalamata olives
- ☐ liquid smoke
- ☐ macaroni
- ☐ noodles (whole-grain; e.g., buckwheat)
- ☐ nuts (optional)
- ☐ oats (instant and rolled)
- ☐ pizza sauce or marinara sauce (optional)
- ☐ raisins/dates
- ☐ roasted red peppers (in water, *not* oil)
- ☐ smooth peanut butter
- ☐ tofu (soft, shelf-stable; e.g., Mori-Nu)
- ☐ vegetable broth (low sodium)
- ☐ vinegar

spices and dry herbs

- [ ] allspice
- [ ] bay leaves
- [ ] black pepper
- [ ] black salt
- [ ] cayenne pepper
- [ ] chili powder
- [ ] chipotle powder
- [ ] curry powder (mild)
- [ ] dried oregano
- [ ] garam masala
- [ ] garlic powder (granulated)
- [ ] ground cinnamon
- [ ] ground coriander
- [ ] ground cumin
- [ ] ground ginger
- [ ] ground nutmeg
- [ ] Italian seasoning
- [ ] nutritional yeast
- [ ] onion flakes
- [ ] onion powder (granulated)
- [ ] paprika (regular and smoked)
- [ ] poultry seasoning
  (granulated, *not* powdered)
- [ ] pumpkin pie spice
- [ ] red pepper flakes
- [ ] rubbed sage (*not* powdered)
- [ ] salt
- [ ] taco seasoning (packet)
- [ ] Thai green curry paste (jar)
- [ ] Thai red curry paste (jar)
- [ ] turmeric

baking

- [ ] agave nectar (optional)
- [ ] baking powder
- [ ] baking soda
- [ ] banana extract (optional)
- [ ] brown sugar
- [ ] chocolate chips (vegan)
- [ ] chocolate extract (optional)
- [ ] confectioner's sugar
- [ ] cornmeal
- [ ] cornstarch or arrowroot
- [ ] mint or peppermint extract
- [ ] molasses (*not* blackstrap)
- [ ] pure maple syrup
- [ ] raw sugar
- [ ] unsweetened cocoa
- [ ] vanilla extract
- [ ] vital wheat gluten*
- [ ] white whole-wheat flour*
- [ ] whole-wheat pastry flour (optional)*

*gluten-free substitutes

- [ ] gluten-free all-purpose flour blend
- [ ] Orgran's Gluten Free Gluten
  Substitute
- [ ] gluten-free tamari

soy-free substitutes

- [ ] chickpea miso
- [ ] coconut aminos

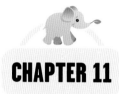

CHAPTER 11

recipes

how to use the icons in this book

| GF | SF |

GLUTEN-FREE Recipes that don't require wheat or barley. I can't vouch for every ingredient, though, so if you have an allergy or sensitivity, please make sure every ingredient you use is certified gluten-free. For example, while oats themselves do not contain gluten, they may be cross-contaminated. Recipes with an asterisk next to the icon can be made gluten-free with simple substitutions. For example, use gluten-free tamari or coconut aminos in place of soy sauce. In non-baking recipes, rice flour is a fairly good replacement for whole-wheat flour.

SOY-FREE Recipes that don't require tofu or tempeh. Recipes with an asterisk next to the icon can be made soy-free with simple substitutions. For example, use coconut aminos in place of soy sauce, chickpea miso when miso is called for, and almond milk instead of soy milk.

> *Nutritional information for each recipe was computed using caloriecount.com. Each analysis provided is per serving. Unless otherwise noted, optional ingredients are not included, and when a recipe calls for multiple amounts (e.g., three to four garlic cloves), the lesser amount is computed. For nondairy milk, unsweetened almond milk was used in the calculation. Breads and buns are not included in the nutritional analysis (see packaging for that information). Sodium content is also not included because values are significantly different between brands and because the calculator tools have too much discrepancy with sodium values to provide a safe and reliable estimate.*

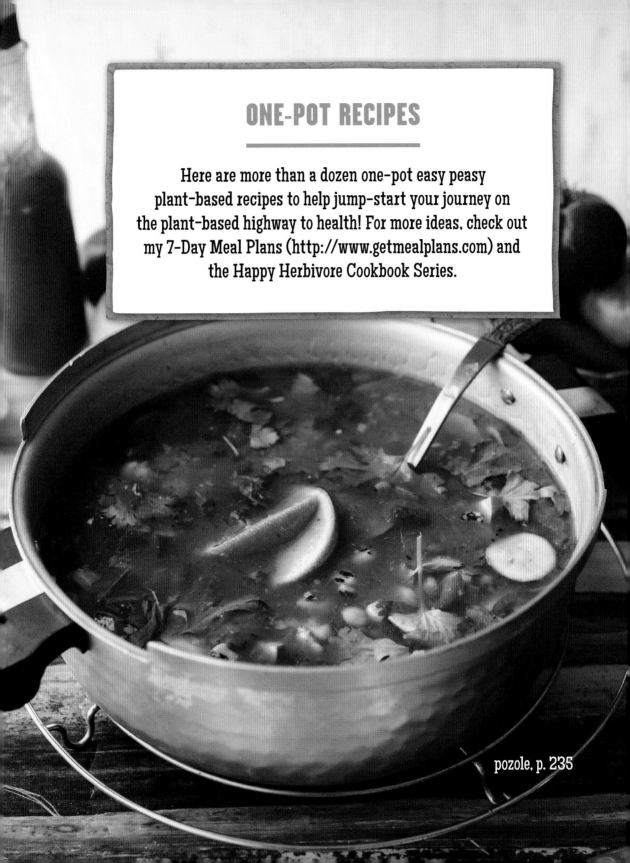

ONE-POT RECIPES

Here are more than a dozen one-pot easy peasy plant-based recipes to help jump-start your journey on the plant-based highway to health! For more ideas, check out my 7-Day Meal Plans (http://www.getmealplans.com) and the Happy Herbivore Cookbook Series.

pozole, p. 235

bean soup

SERVES 1–2 | **GF** | **SF** | Before my dad went plant-based, he loved Campbell's Bean and Bacon soup. For his sixty-eighth birthday, I figured out how to make a copycat version.

½ c vegetable broth, divided
1 small onion, diced
1 carrot, diced
1 celery stalk, sliced
2 bay leaves
1 15-oz can white beans, undrained
½ tsp smoked paprika
¼ tsp maple syrup
1 tsp tomato paste
Liquid smoke (optional)

1. Sauté onion, carrot, celery, and bay leaves in ¼ cup broth. When the broth evaporates, add remaining broth. Continue to cook until everything is really soft. Remove bay leaves.

2. Use immersion blender (and a little water as needed) to purée until it's silky smooth.

3. Add beans, including their liquid, and use an immersion blender again to purée, but leaving some half beans.

4. Stir in paprika, maple syrup, and tomato paste. Add salt and pepper to taste, plus a drop (or two) liquid smoke (use very, very little!), more smoked paprika, or tomato paste (or ketchup for a hint of sweetness) as desired.

If using a regular blender: Transfer sautéed vegetable mix to blender and add water as necessary to purée (using the bare minimum). Reserve ½ cup beans, and put remaining beans and liquid in blender and purée. Return to pot, mix in leftover beans, and add remaining ingredients. Use a potato masher to mash up the beans into half beans, then adjust seasonings to taste.

> **PER SERVING (SERVING 2):** 230 calories, 1.9g fat, 40.1g carbohydrates, 12.4g fiber, 4.1g sugars, 13.2g protein

"beef" and broccoli

SERVES 1–2 | **GF*** | **SF*** | There isn't any beef in this recipe, or broccoli for that matter (since I'm allergic to broccoli, I use green bell pepper). Yet, to me this meal tastes exactly like the "beef and broccoli" dish you order from a Chinese takeout stand, hence the name. This is a terrific weeknight meal. Serve over rice.

1 large portobello mushroom, de-stemmed and diced

2 cups No-Beef Broth, divided (p. 238)

1 small onion, diced

2–3 garlic cloves, minced

2–3 tsp fresh ginger, minced

2 tbsp ketchup

½ tsp mild curry powder

1 tsp rice vinegar

1 green bell pepper, seeded and sliced (or broccoli)

Asian hot sauce (optional)

1 tsp cornstarch mixed in 1 tbsp water

CHEF'S NOTE: If you're in a hurry, mix 2 cups water with 2 tbsp soy sauce and 2 tbsp nutritional yeast instead of making the broth.

1. Line skillet with about ½ cup broth and sauté mushrooms until soft, brown, and juicy (most of the liquid should be absorbed during cooking; add more if necessary). Set aside on a plate.

2. Reline skillet with another ½ cup broth and sauté onions, garlic, and ginger for a few minutes, until very fragrant and onion is translucent.

3. Add ketchup, curry, vinegar, and bell pepper, plus more broth as needed, and continue to cook until bell peppers are very soft and darker in color.

4. Add black pepper to taste if desired.

5. Stir in cooked mushrooms. Add broth if necessary—you want some liquid, but don't add too much or it will dilute the sauce.

6. Add hot sauce to taste (I do about ½ tsp) and more curry if desired, and stir to combine.

7. Once mushrooms are warm (about a minute), add cornstarch slurry and reduce heat slightly. Continue to stir and let the sauce thicken.

8. Garnish with sliced green onion or sesame seeds if desired and serve over prepared rice.

> **PER SERVING (SERVING 1):** 240 calories, 1.9g fat, 43.2g carbohydrates, 11.2g fiber, 15.4g sugars, 17.4g protein

* THERE IS SOY SAUCE IN THE NO-BEEF BROTH MIX. SEE P. 238 FOR GF AND SF ALTERNATIVES IN THAT RECIPE.

belize bean quesadillas

SERVES 1-2 | **GF** | **SF** | When my husband and I were in Belize, he became obsessed with black bean and banana quesadillas (basically, black beans and bananas in a tortilla, then warmed). He ate them every single day, sometimes twice a day, asking for them even at breakfast. (We'd seen "Banana Quesadillas" on the menu made from cheese and bananas. Scott asked for beans instead of cheese and the rest is history.) I know it sounds a bit odd, but they're really good!

1 small onion, diced

2-3 garlic cloves, minced

1 small jalapeño, seeded and minced (optional)

1 tsp chili powder

½ tsp ground cumin

Light dash of paprika

Very light dash of cinnamon

1 15-oz can black beans, undrained

1 lime, juiced and zested

1-2 ripe bananas

FOR THE BEANS:

1. Line a skillet with a thin layer of water and sauté onion, garlic, and jalapeño (if using) over high heat until onion is translucent and most of the water has cooked off, or about 2 minutes.

2. Add chili powder, cumin, a light dash of paprika, and a very light dash of cinnamon, stirring to coat everything. Continue to cook for about a minute, or until fragrant and most of the liquid has cooked off.

3. Add beans (with their liquid) and stir to combine. Reduce heat to low and mash beans well with a fork or potato masher a few times. You still want some whole and half beans and not a refried consistency. It will look very soupy; don't be alarmed.

4. Crank the heat to high and bring to a boil. Once boiling, reduce heat to medium-high and cook for 10 minutes. If it's popping, cover for a few minutes or until it cools down and stops popping. Stir the beans every minute or so, taking care to scrape the bottom and lift the beans. After 10 minutes, the mixture should have significantly reduced. It may still be a little soupy, which is all right—it will thicken as it cools—but if it's really soupy, cook longer.

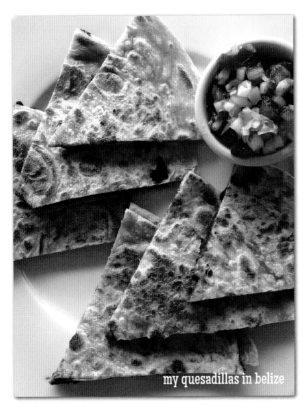
my quesadillas in belize

5. Add lime juice (and zest) to taste, plus hot sauce (optional).

FOR THE BANANAS:

You can either mash them up into the beans or "fry" slices (see note) and add on top. Spread into your tortilla and dry fry the quesadilla for a few minutes.

PER SERVING (WITH 1 BANANA): 280 calories, 2.4g fat, 53.9g carbohydrates, 14.3g fiber, 9.4g sugars, 14.1g protein

PER SERVING (WITH 2 BANANAS): 333 calories, 2.6g fat, 67.3g carbohydrates, 15.9g fiber, 16.6g sugars, 14.7g protein

*THE RECIPE IS GLUTEN-FREE AS LONG AS YOU USE A GF TORTILLA SUCH AS BROWN RICE OR CORN.

CHEF'S NOTES:
- In Belize, they use habanero-based hot sauce.
- To "fry" bananas, peel & slice into 1-inch chunks, then slice each chunk in half lengthwise (down the center of the banana). Heat a nonstick skillet over high heat. Place slimy insides facedown on the skillet, one at a time, in a row. Flip the bananas over (in the same order you put them down originally) so each piece "fries" for 1-2 minutes on both sides.

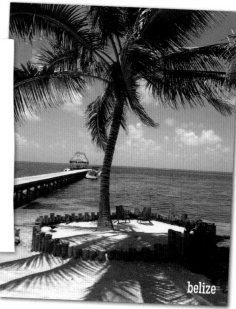
belize

butternut and pea curry

SERVES 1 | **GF** | **SF** | A quick and easy fall weeknight recipe.

1¼ c vegetable broth, divided
1 small onion, diced
3 garlic cloves, minced
    Red pepper flakes (optional)
2½ c butternut squash, cubed
1½ tbsp mild curry powder
½ c frozen peas
1 tsp cornstarch
½–1 tsp brown sugar
¼ c nondairy milk

CHEF'S NOTE: Some of my testers liked this with sweet potatoes, but everyone preferred butternut.

1. Line wide skillet with ¼ cup broth. Sauté onions and garlic (and red pepper flakes, if using—add as desired for heat) until onions are translucent and liquid has mostly or entirely evaporated.

2. Add butternut, curry, and remaining 1 cup broth. Cover and bring to a boil.

3. Reduce to simmer and cook until butternut is just fork tender, about 5-7 minutes. Add peas and stir.

4. Continue to cook a few more minutes, until peas are soft and butternut has softened, but is not falling apart or mushy.

5. Whisk cornstarch and sugar into nondairy milk and pour over dish. Stir, then cook for another minute, allowing the sauce to thicken slightly.

6. Cover and let sit for a few minutes. Once it has cooled (still warm but not piping hot), taste, adding more curry or sugar to taste (reheat briefly if you add more).

7. Serve over rice or quinoa.

PER SERVING: 363 calories, 4.3g fat, 72.4g carbohydrates, 16.4g fiber, 16.9g sugars, 16.4g protein

caribbean ragout

SERVES 2 | **GF** | **SF** | Instead of pasta and marinara sauce, we have rice and a Caribbean-inspired black bean sauce. Quick, easy, and delicious!

Vegetable broth, as needed

½ small onion, diced

3–4 garlic cloves, minced

1 red bell pepper, seeded and diced

2–4 green onions, sliced

½ c pineapple, diced

¼ c cilantro, divided

¾ tsp chili powder

½ tsp ground cumin

¼ tsp ground ginger

Dash of paprika (regular or smoked)

Dash of cinnamon

2–3 tbsp canned green chilies

1 15-oz can black beans (drained and rinsed, unless no salt added)

1 small lime, juiced

Green tabasco hot sauce (optional)

1. Line a skillet with a thin layer of broth. Sauté onion and garlic until onion is translucent.

2. Add pepper, more broth, and green onions (reserving some dark green parts for garnish), and stir. Cook for a minute or so.

3. Add pineapple, half the cilantro, and the seasonings, stirring to combine. Cook for a minute or so.

4. Add green chilies, beans, and more vegetable broth. Cover and simmer for a few minutes, until bell peppers and pineapple are really tender (about 5 minutes).

5. Use a potato masher to mash up some of the mixture (if desired for a thicker sauce). If it gets too dry, add more broth.

6. Add lime juice to taste, plus salt if desired.

7. Let flavors blend for 5 minutes before serving. Top with remaining cilantro and green onion. Serve over rice and drizzle with green hot sauce if desired.

PER SERVING: 272 calories, 2.3g fat, 49.8g carbohydrates, 13.4g fiber, 10.6g sugars, 14.2g protein

"cheater" tofu lettuce wraps

SERVES 2 | **GF*** | Right after I went vegetarian, I discovered the Tofu Lettuce Wraps at P. F. Chang's. It was a lifesaver in some ways because P. F. Chang's was already a favorite restaurant among my omnivore friends, who thought my new vegetarianism was strange. (Which I guess wasn't so strange after all when they kept helping themselves to my order!) Now I make my own lighter version at home.

1 15-oz block extra-firm tofu

2 tbsp vegetable broth

1 shallot, minced

2 tsp fresh ginger, minced

4 garlic cloves, minced

2 tbsp low-sodium soy sauce

1 tbsp peanut butter

1 tbsp rice vinegar

1–3 tsp Asian hot sauce (i.e., sriracha)

1 tbsp sweet red chili sauce

1 tbsp hoisin sauce

1 tsp Vegan Worcestershire Sauce (p. 240)

1 tbsp ketchup

Green onions, sliced

Lettuce wraps

1. Press the tofu (see note).

2. Line a skillet with a very thin layer of broth and sauté shallot, fresh ginger, and garlic until fragrant and water has evaporated.

3. Whisk soy sauce, remaining broth, peanut butter, vinegar, hot sauce, sweet red chili sauce, hoisin sauce, Worcestershire sauce, and ketchup together in a small bowl. Meanwhile, add tofu to a skillet and break into big chunks with a spatula. Cook, stirring to incorporate everything. Add sauce and stir to combine.

4. Continue to cook a few minutes, until sauce absorbs into tofu.

5. Let cool almost to room temperature. Add more hoisin, hot sauce, or peanut butter as desired.

6. Garnish with green onions and spoon into lettuce wraps. Should be served just barely warmer than room temperature.

PER SERVING (JUST TOFU MIXTURE):
277 calories, 13.4g fat, 21.6g carbohydrates, 3.1g fiber, 10g sugars, 21.5g protein

CHEF'S NOTE: Press the tofu by wrapping the tofu in a clean kitchen cloth and placing between two cutting boards. Place a large, heavy object on the top board. Allow to rest for 20 minutes, forcing excess water out of the tofu.

*REPLACE SOY SAUCE WITH TAMARI TO MAKE THIS RECIPE GLUTEN-FREE.

indian lentils & cabbage

SERVES 2–3 | **GF** | **SF** | I'm always looking for more ways to bring cabbage into my diet, and pairing it with lentils and Indian spices is a nice twist. To speed this dish up, cook lentils in a small pot while you cook the cabbage.

½ c red lentils

1 c vegetable broth

1 small onion, diced

3 garlic cloves, minced

2–3 tsp fresh ginger, minced

Red pepper flakes or cayenne pepper (optional)

1 tsp yellow mustard

½ tsp ground cumin

1 small head cabbage, sliced thin

Few dashes of turmeric

¼ c tomato sauce

Few dashes of garam masala

1 tomato, diced (optional)

CHEF'S NOTE: My recipe testers had luck with this dish in the slow cooker on low.

1. In a large pot, combine lentils with 1 cup water. Cover and bring to a boil.

2. Reduce heat to low and simmer for 7–10 minutes, or until lentils are soft and have turned orange, and the water has evaporated. (If lentils are not done or crunchy, add more water and cook a bit longer.) Scoop them into a small bowl or dish.

3. Line your large pot with a thin layer of broth. Sauté onion, garlic, and ginger over high heat until onions are translucent, adding splashes of broth as necessary.

4. Add red pepper flakes or cayenne pepper (as desired), mustard, cumin, and cabbage.

5. Continue to cook, stirring often, until cabbage starts to soften, adding more broth as necessary.

6. Add a few dashes of turmeric and continue to stir and cook.

7. Once cabbage is soft, add tomato sauce and a few dashes of garam masala. Continue to cook and stir.

8. Turn off heat, add cooked lentils and tomato (if using), and stir to combine. Add another dash or so of garam masala, to taste, plus salt and pepper if desired.

9. Let dish cool and allow flavors to meld for a few minutes, then serve.

PER SERVING (SERVING 2): 304 calories, 1.3g fat, 59.5g carbohydrates, 25.5g fiber, 15.7g sugars, 18.4g protein.

lemon takeout chickpeas

SERVES 2-3 | **GF*** | **SF*** | Before I was plant-based, I loved ordering Chinese lemon chicken takeout. It was sweet more than lemony, and I missed those flavors until I realized how easy they were to capture with my favorite "chicken" replacement (chickpeas) and pineapple! (Yes, pineapple! That was the secret—not lemon!) Serve over rice with a side of broccoli for a complete meal.

2 c frozen pineapple

½ tsp cornstarch

Vegetable broth, as needed

2 garlic cloves, minced

2 tsp fresh ginger, minced

½ red bell pepper, seeded and diced

1 tsp rice vinegar

1 tbsp low-sodium soy sauce

1 tbsp sweet red chili sauce

1 15-oz can chickpeas, drained and rinsed

2 green onions, sliced

1 lemon, juiced

1. Thaw frozen pineapple in a bowl (to catch juices).

2. Whisk cornstarch into 2 tbsp water and set aside.

3. Line a skillet with a thin layer of broth and sauté garlic, ginger, and bell pepper until fragrant, liquid has evaporated, and bell peppers have softened.

4. Add a tiny splash of rice vinegar to help scrape up bits, then add pineapple with juice, soy sauce, sweet red chili sauce, chickpeas, and green onions (reserving some for garnish), plus a splash of broth if necessary.

5. Continue to cook, stirring to incorporate.

6. Add cornstarch mix and let thicken over low heat.

7. Turn off heat and add half the lemon juice. Stir and let cool slightly.

8. Taste, adding more lemon juice as desired. Garnish with remaining green onions.

CHEF'S NOTE: Add lemon zest for a stronger lemon taste.

> **PER SERVING (SERVING 2):** 366 calories, 2.1g fat, 70.5g carbohydrates, 11.6g fiber, 21.8g sugars, 14.9g protein

* REPLACE SOY SAUCE WITH TAMARI TO MAKE THIS RECIPE GLUTEN-FREE, OR WITH COCONUT AMINOS TO MAKE IT SOY-FREE.

mexican quinoa

SERVES 1 | **GF** | **SF** | This is my "fix it and forget it" quinoa dish.

¼ c quinoa

½–¾ c vegetable broth

¼ c canned green chilies

½ jalapeño (optional)

1 tsp chili powder

½ tsp ground cumin

½ tsp oregano

½ tsp onion powder

½ tsp garlic powder

Dash of cayenne pepper (optional)

½ c frozen fire-roasted corn

1 tomato, diced

2 tbsp tomato sauce

½ small lime

1 green onion, sliced

3 tbsp cilantro

½ c black beans, cooked or canned, rinsed

1. In a small saucepan, combine quinoa, ½ cup broth, chilies, jalapeño, and spices. Stir to combine.

2. Cover, bring to a boil, then reduce to low and simmer until quinoa is fluffy and broth has evaporated.

3. Add corn, tomato, and tomato sauce and stir to combine. Cook over low heat, adding a splash or two of broth as necessary, until tomatoes are softer and corn is cooked.

4. Squeeze lime and stir in juice.

5. Stir in green onion and cilantro.

6. Stir in black beans, then add salt and pepper to taste and more cayenne or hot sauce (if desired).

> **PER SERVING:** 391 calories, 4.9g fat, 73.6g carbohydrates, 13.7g fiber, 8.9g sugars, 16.9g protein

moroccan carrot soup

SERVES 1–2 | **GF** | **SF** | This Moroccan spiced carrot soup is blended with beans, which gives it a nice creamy element.

1¼ c vegetable broth
1 small onion, diced
2–3 garlic cloves, minced
1–2 carrots, sliced
1 15-oz can white beans, drained and rinsed
Ras el hanout, to taste (see Chef's Note)

1. Line a pot with a thin layer of broth and sauté onion, garlic, and carrots (use 2 carrots for a stronger carrot flavor) until onions are translucent and carrots are fork tender.

2. Transfer to a blender (or use an immersion blender), with beans and purée, adding more broth as necessary (I usually add about 1 cup) until it's a creamy soup consistency.

3. Return to the pot and heat over low until warm.

4. Add ras el hanout to taste (I typically add just a few light dashes, about ⅛ tsp, but add as much as you like).

CHEF'S NOTE: Ras el hanout is a North African spice blend, made from common spices we all have on hand, such as ginger, coriander, cinnamon, ground pepper, turmeric, nutmeg, and allspice (the name literally translates to "head of the shop," implying it is a mixture of the best spices the seller has to offer). Sometimes it's sold under the name "Moroccan Spices." If your local supermarket or spice shop doesn't carry it, you can easily find a recipe online.

> **PER SERVING (USING 2 CARROTS, SERVING 2):**
> 233 calories, 1.8g fat, 41g carbohydrates, 12g fiber, 3.5g sugars, 13.2g protein

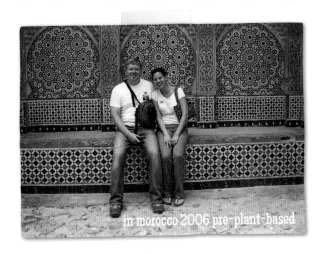

in morocco 2006 pre-plant-based

moroccan chickpeas

SERVES 2 | **GF** | **SF** | Moroccan spices and flavorings are definitely something I've warmed up to in the last year or so. (Just add "Moroccan" to the long list of cuisines I've discovered and loved since going plant-based!) If you've ever had the classic dish Moroccan meatballs, the flavorings here will be familiar to you. And, true to Moroccan cuisine, I like to serve these chickpeas over whole-wheat couscous.

1 28-oz can diced fire-roasted tomatoes

1 onion, diced

3–4 garlic cloves, minced

Vegetable broth, as needed

10–12 fresh mint leaves, divided

¼ c cilantro, divided

1–3 tsp ras el hanout (see Chef's Note, previous page)

¼ tsp ground cumin

Cinnamon

¼ tsp paprika (regular or smoked)

1 15-oz can chickpeas, drained and rinsed

1 large zucchini, cut into half moons

Agave nectar or sugar (optional)

1. Drain tomato juices into a skillet. Add onions, garlic, and broth as needed to create a thin layer of liquid. Sauté until onions are translucent.

2. Add half the mint and cilantro, 1 tsp ras el hanout, cumin, a few light dashes of cinnamon, paprika (or try smoked paprika!), chickpeas, and tomatoes. Cover and bring to a boil.

3. Simmer for 5 minutes.

4. Stir and add zucchini. Continue to simmer until zucchini is tender.

5. Stir in remaining cilantro and mint, plus a little sugar or agave (about 1–2 tsp) if your tomatoes are too acidic.

6. Let rest 5 minutes. Add additional ras el hanout to taste and serve.

> **PER SERVING:** 355 calories, 2.8g fat, 64.9g carbohydrates, 16g fiber, 16.6g sugars, 18g protein

mushroom
& potato soup

SERVES 1–2 | **GF**∗ | **SF**∗ | This soup reminds me of beef stew, though it's not necessarily a plant-based rendition of beef stew. I love making it during the cold months and serving it with biscuits or pouring it over mashed potatoes or cooked grains.

3–4 c No-Beef Broth (p. 238)

1 onion, diced

1 1-inch piece ginger, peeled but left intact

2 carrots, sliced

2 bay leaves

1–2 celery stalks, sliced

1½ c mushrooms, sliced

½ sprig fresh rosemary

1 potato, diced

1. Line a large pot with 1 cup broth. Combine onion, ginger, and carrots, and bring to a boil.

2. Once carrots start to become fork tender and onion turns translucent, add bay leaves, celery, and mushrooms plus 1 cup broth and rosemary. Cover, bring to a boil again, and simmer until mushrooms are soft (but not mushy).

3. Scoop out and discard ginger, then add potato and 1 cup broth. Cover, bring to a boil again, then reduce to low.

4. Simmer until broth is thick and potatoes are tender. If it gets too thin, add more broth or water.

5. Remove bay leaves. Season with salt and pepper as desired.

CHEF'S NOTE: For a saucier dish, add a little Vegan Worcestershire Sauce (p. 240) to taste.

PER SERVING (SERVING 2): 173 calories, 1g fat, 34g carbohydrates, 8.1g fiber, 7.2g sugars, 10.7g protein

∗ FOR GLUTEN-FREE USE TAMARI INSTEAD OF SOY SAUCE IN THE BROTH. FOR SOY-FREE, USE COCONUT AMINOS.

pozole (pictured on page 221)

SERVES 3-4 | **GF** | **SF** | Right before I started writing this book, I asked my fans (called "Herbies") on Facebook what recipe they'd like me to re-create that I haven't already. Pozole, a traditional pre-Columbian soup from Mexico, was the top request! The secret to good pozole is a very flavorful broth—don't be shy with your cilantro or lime!

2 c vegetable broth
1 tsp ground cumin
1 medium onion, diced
4 garlic cloves, minced
1 tsp dried oregano
2-3 very light dashes of ground cloves
½ c cilantro
⅓ c salsa verde (green salsa)
1 zucchini (or 2 small ones), sliced
1 large tomato, sliced, with juices
½ c fire-roasted frozen corn
1 c hominy
1 lime, juiced
Dash of chipotle pepper (optional)
Dash of smoked paprika (optional)

1. Line a large pot with a thin layer of broth (about ¼ cup). Add cumin, onion, and garlic. Sauté until onion is translucent.

2. Add oregano, 2–3 very light dashes of cloves, ¼ cup broth, ¼ cup cilantro, and salsa. Stir to combine and cook for a minute or so.

3. Add zucchini, reduce heat, and continue to cook, until zucchini is just fork tender, or about 2 minutes.

4. Add tomato with juices, remaining broth, 1 cup water, and corn. Continue to simmer for a minute, or until corn is warm.

5. Turn off heat and stir in hominy. Add another 2–4 tbsp cilantro.

6. After a few minutes, add the juice of half the lime. Taste, adding more salsa or lime if desired.

PER SERVING (SERVING 3): 130 calories, 1.3g fat, 28g carbohydrates, 5.2g fat, 7.9g sugars, 4.5g protein

CHEF'S NOTES:

• Hominy hides in a can in the Mexican section of your supermarket, usually on the bottom shelf.

• For a smoky heat, add chipotle or adobo. For just a smoky element, add smoked paprika.

southwestern loaf

SERVES 4 (1 LOAF) | **GF** | **SF** | This loaf doesn't taste like "meatloaf," but it's delicious in its own right. Serve with chipotle ketchup, corn, sweet potatoes, and greens for a colorful (fiesta!) meal.

2 15-oz cans black beans, drained and rinsed

4 oz diced green chilies

¼ c ketchup

2 tbsp yellow mustard

1 tsp onion powder

1 tsp garlic powder

¼ c salsa (spicy or medium)

⅓ c frozen corn

Hot sauce or cayenne (optional)

1 c instant oats

1. Preheat oven to 350°F and set aside a standard 8-inch metal loaf pan.

2. Mash the beans with a fork (or pulse in a food processor) so no whole beans are left, but so it's still chunky, with some half beans.

3. Transfer to a mixing bowl and add remaining ingredients (except oats) in order, adding hot sauce or cayenne as desired for more heat.

4. Once combined, add oats and combine again.

5. Transfer combined mixture to loaf pan and bake 35–45 minutes, until firmer and crisp on the top (not still wet).

6. Let cool in the pan for 10–20 minutes before serving, if possible (it firms as it cools).

PER SERVING: 282 calories, 3.1g fat, 48.9g carbohydrates, 12.4g fiber, 5.8g sugars, 15.2g protein

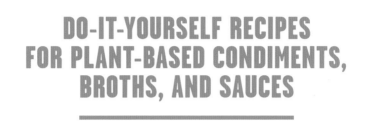

DO-IT-YOURSELF RECIPES FOR PLANT-BASED CONDIMENTS, BROTHS, AND SAUCES

Here are a few of my go-to DIY substitutes for broths, dairy, and condiments! There's no shortage of commercial options, too (see p. 120)!

aj's vegan parmesan, p. 239

no-beef broth

MAKES 1 CUP | **GF*** | **SF*** | This is my DIY version for faux beef broth and it can easily be made gluten- and soy-free.

CHEF'S NOTE: If you use this broth in a soup recipe, add a bay leaf during cooking.

1 tbsp low-sodium soy sauce*
1 tbsp nutritional yeast
½ tsp Vegan Worcestershire Sauce (p. 240)*
¼ tsp onion powder
¼ tsp garlic powder
¼ tsp ground ginger
⅛ tsp black pepper
Salt, to taste

1. In a medium saucepan, whisk all ingredients together with 1 cup water until well combined.
2. Bring to a boil and let simmer for 1 minute.
3. Add salt to taste, if desired.

> **PER SERVING (1 C):** 27 calories, 0.2g fat, 4.3g carbohy-drates, 1.1g fiber, 0.7g sugars, 2.7g protein

*FOR GLUTEN-FREE USE TAMARI INSTEAD OF SOY SAUCE. FOR SOY-FREE, USE COCONUT AMINOS.

no-chicken broth

MAKES 1 CUP | **GF** | **SF** | This is my DIY version for faux chicken broth powder. To make broth, mix 1 tbsp of the powder into 1 cup of warm or hot water.

1⅓ c nutritional yeast
2 tbsp onion powder
1 tbsp garlic powder
1 tsp dried thyme
1 tsp rubbed sage (not powdered)
1 tsp paprika
½ tsp turmeric
¼ tsp celery seed
¼ tsp dried parsley

Combine all ingredients in a mortar and pestle, then grind into a fine powder.

> **PER SERVING (1 TBSP):** 12 calories, 0.1g fat, 1.7g carbo-hydrates, 0.7g fiber, 0g sugars, 1.3g protein

(pictured on page 237)

aj's vegan parmesan

MAKES 1½ CUPS | **GF** | **SF** | If you can't find commercial vegan Parmesan where you live, here is a great alternative recipe by my friend Chef AJ. AJ says, "I've made this with almonds, walnuts, cashews, even Brazil nuts. For those with a nut allergy, use sesame seeds."

1 c nuts
½ c nutritional yeast
Pinch of salt or salt-free seasoning (optional)

1. Put nuts and nutritional yeast in a blender.

2. Add salt or salt-free seasoning (e.g., garlic powder and/or onion powder), if desired.

3. Process until a smooth powder has formed.

4. Store in an airtight container in the fridge for up to a week.

> **PER SERVING (1 TBSP, WITH CASHEWS):** 45 calories, 2.8g fat, 3.4g carbohydrates, 1g fiber, 0g sugars, 2.4g protein

vegan mayo

MAKES 1 CUP | **GF** | I make my own mayo from tofu, but in a pinch vegan yogurt (same amount as the mayo) with a touch of lemon or white vinegar does the trick.

1 12.3-oz pkg tofu (the softer the better)
2-3 tbsp Dijon mustard
2 tsp distilled white vinegar
Fresh lemon and agave, to taste

1. In a blender or small food processor, blend tofu with Dijon and vinegar until smooth and creamy.

2. Add a few drops of lemon juice and a few drops of agave nectar and blend again.

3. Taste and add more lemon, agave, or Dijon as needed or desired. Chill until you're ready to use.

> **PER SERVING (1 TBSP):** 9 calories, 0.2g fat, 0.3g carbohydrates, 0g fiber, 0g sugars, 1.6g protein

vegan worcestershire sauce

MAKES 1 CUP | **GF*** | **SF*** | Most commercial Worcestershire sauces contain anchovies, although there are a few vegetarian brands on the market. While nothing beats the ease of bottled sauce, this DIY recipe is allergen-free and very inexpensive to make.

6 tbsp apple cider vinegar

2 tbsp low-sodium soy sauce

1 tbsp brown sugar or 1 tsp molasses (*not* blackstrap)

2 tsp prepared mustard (any)

¼ tsp onion powder

¼ tsp garlic powder

¼ tsp cinnamon

Light dash of cayenne pepper or chili powder

Light dash of allspice or ground cloves

1. Whisk all ingredients together with ¼ cup water until well combined.

2. Add salt if desired.

3. Store in an airtight container in the fridge.

PER SERVING (1 TSP): 2 calories, 0g fat, 0.4g carbohydrates, 0g fiber, 0g sugars, 0.1g protein

* FOR GLUTEN-FREE USE TAMARI INSTEAD OF SOY SAUCE. FOR SOY-FREE, USE COCONUT AMINOS.

golden dressing

MAKES ABOUT ½ CUP | **GF** | **SF*** | This recipe visits us from *Happy Herbivore Light & Lean* and is my favorite dressing to serve. My omni friends practically drink it, they love it so much. Add more miso for a miso dressing, more Dijon for a spicy or tangy dressing, more lemon for a lemony dressing, and so on. I also like to substitute peanut butter or tahini for the miso on occasion.

¼ c cold water

¼ c nutritional yeast

1–2 tbsp Dijon mustard

1 tbsp pure maple syrup or 1–2 dates

½ lemon, skin removed and seeded

1 tbsp yellow miso (see note)

1. Combine all ingredients in a blender and blend until smooth and creamy, adding more water if you like a thinner dressing (note: this dressing thickens as it chills in the fridge).

2. Taste, adding more nutritional yeast, Dijon, maple syrup (or dates), lemon, or miso as desired.

> **PER SERVING (1 TSP, WITH MISO):** 21 calories, 0.3g fat, 3.3g carbohydrates, 1g fiber, 1.2g sugars, 1.8g protein
>
> **PER SERVING (1 TSP, WITH PEANUT BUTTER):** 25 calories, 0.9g fat, 3.2g carbohydrates, 1g fiber, 1.2g sugars, 1.9g protein

* FOR SOY-FREE USE CHICKPEA-BASED MISO.

CHEF'S NOTE: I use yellow miso, but white, red, or chickpea miso should also work. Do not use brown miso.

creamy cajun mustard

MAKES ⅓ CUP | **GF*** | **SF*** | You can find commercial creamy Cajun mustard in Louisiana, but I prefer making it myself so it's always available and I can adjust the heat to my preferences.

3 tbsp Dijon mustard

½ tsp Vegan Worcestershire Sauce (p. 240)*

½ tsp hot sauce

1 tsp molasses (*not* blackstrap)

1 tbsp Vegan Mayo (p. 239) or plain vegan yogurt*

¼ tsp Cajun seasoning

1. Combine all ingredients, adding more Cajun Seasoning if you like.

2. If your Dijon is too strong, you can add a bit more mayo to tone it down. You can also add a touch more molasses for a sweeter mustard.

> **PER SERVING (1 TBSP):** 12 calories, 0.4g fat, 1.8g carbohydrates, 0g fiber, 1.1g sugars, 0.6g protein

vegan sour cream

MAKES 1 CUP | **GF** | Quick and easy and so healthy!

VARIATION » LIME CRÈME: Use lime juice instead of lemon juice and add 1½ tbsp chopped cilantro.

1 12.3-oz pkg Mori-Nu firm tofu

2–4 tbsp fresh lemon juice

½ tsp distilled white vinegar

⅛ tsp fine salt

1 tsp dry mustard powder

Agave nectar, to taste

Light dash of garlic powder

1 tsp dried or fresh dill (optional)

1. Combine tofu with 2 tbsp lemon juice, vinegar, a pinch of salt, mustard powder, a few drops of agave, and garlic powder, and blend until smooth and creamy.

2. Taste and add more lemon and/or agave if necessary or desired. Stir in dill before serving if using.

> **PER SERVING (1 TBSP):** 13 calories, 0.2g fat, 1.4g carbohydrates, 0g fiber, 1.1g sugars, 1.6g protein

everyday mushroom gravy

MAKES 1 CUP |**GF***|**SF***| You might remember this gravy recipe from *Everyday Happy Herbivore*. It's so great, versatile, and low calorie that I had to include it again!

2 tbsp low-sodium soy sauce

2 tbsp nutritional yeast, divided

¼ tsp granulated onion powder

¼ tsp granulated garlic powder

¼ tsp ground ginger

8 oz white or brown mushrooms, sliced

Italian seasoning

½ c nondairy milk

2 tbsp cornstarch

Dash of ground nutmeg (optional)

CHEF'S NOTE: For a smoky-flavored gravy, substitute smoked paprika for the ground nutmeg, and add more to taste.

1. In a skillet, whisk 1 cup water with soy sauce, 1 tbsp of nutritional yeast, onion powder, garlic powder, and ground ginger. Bring to a boil and add mushrooms, sprinkling them generously with Italian seasoning (a good 10 shakes).

2. Continue to sauté over medium-high heat until the mushrooms are brown and soft, about 3 minutes. Meanwhile whisk nondairy milk with cornstarch and remaining 1 tbsp of nutritional yeast. Add a very light dash of ground nutmeg, if desired. Pour over mushrooms, stirring to combine.

3. Reduce heat to low and continue to cook until thick and gravylike, about 5 minutes. Add black pepper to taste (I like it really peppery) and a few more shakes of Italian seasoning unless you were very generous before. Taste again, adding a pinch of salt if necessary.

4. Set aside for a few minutes before serving to let the flavors merge.

> **PER SERVING (ABOUT ¼ CUP):** 60 calories, 1.4g fat, 8.9g carbohydrates, 1.4g fiber, 1.2g sugars, 5.6g protein

*FOR GLUTEN-FREE USE TAMARI INSTEAD OF SOY SAUCE. FOR SOY-FREE, USE COCONUT AMINOS.

ketchup

MAKES 1 TBSP |**GF**|**SF**| I'll be straight with you: Homemade ketchup doesn't exactly taste like Heinz ketchup, but it's delicious in its own right and so much healthier. Less salt, less sugar, no high-fructose corn syrup, and no mystery ingredients! (You'll warm up to homemade ketchup, I promise!)

1½ tbsp tomato paste

1–2 tbsp apple cider vinegar

2 tbsp unsweetened applesauce

1 tsp onion powder

1 tsp garlic powder

Light dash allspice

Pinch brown sugar (1 tsp or less)

2 tbsp tomato sauce

Salt, to taste

1. Whisk all ingredients together, adding more tomato sauce or applesauce as necessary to achieve the right consistency and texture.

> **PER SERVING (1 TBSP):** 8 calories, 0g fat, 1.8g carbohydrates, 0g fiber, 1.2g sugars, 0.3g protein

CHEF'S NOTE: I find some vinegars are stronger than others. Start with 1 tbsp, but expect to increase to a total of 1½–2 tbsp. If you like a vinegary ketchup, 2 tbsp should be more than enough. Also, be careful with the allspice—it's potent! A little goes a long way.

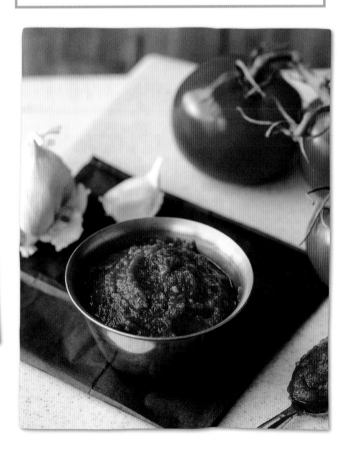

"honey" mustard

MAKES 2 TBSP | **GF** | **SF** | This honey mustard has a slight kick to it. It's great as a dipping sauce, condiment, or salad dressing. I keep a big batch of it in an airtight container in my fridge, but it takes seconds to whip up when you need it.

1 tbsp Dijon mustard
1 tbsp agave nectar
Hot sauce, to taste
Dash of ground ginger

1. In a small bowl, whisk Dijon and agave nectar together.

2. Add a few drops of hot sauce (to your taste) plus a dash or two of ground ginger; mix again.

3. Taste, adjusting agave, mustard, or hot sauce as needed.

PER SERVING (1 TBSP): 38 calories, 0.3 fat, 9.2g carbohydrates, 0g fiber, 8.7g sugars, 0.4g protein

quick queso sauce

MAKES 1 CUP | **GF*** | **SF** | It's okay to go at this sauce with a spoon. I won't judge. It's also great with nachos, burritos, enchiladas, or inside a black bean quesadilla.

1 c nondairy milk
⅓ c nutritional yeast
2 tbsp whole-wheat flour
1 tsp onion powder (granulated)
½ tsp garlic powder (granulated)
½ tsp ground cumin
¼ tsp paprika
¼ tsp chili powder or cayenne (optional)
¼–⅓ c salsa

Whisk all ingredients together in a saucepan. Bring to a boil over medium heat, stirring often until thick. Serve immediately.

PER SERVING (¼ C). 45 calories, 0.8g fat, 6.2g carbohydrates, 1.6g fiber, 1.8g sugars, 4g protein

* USE A GLUTEN-FREE FLOUR SUCH AS BROWN RICE INSTEAD OF WHOLE-WHEAT.

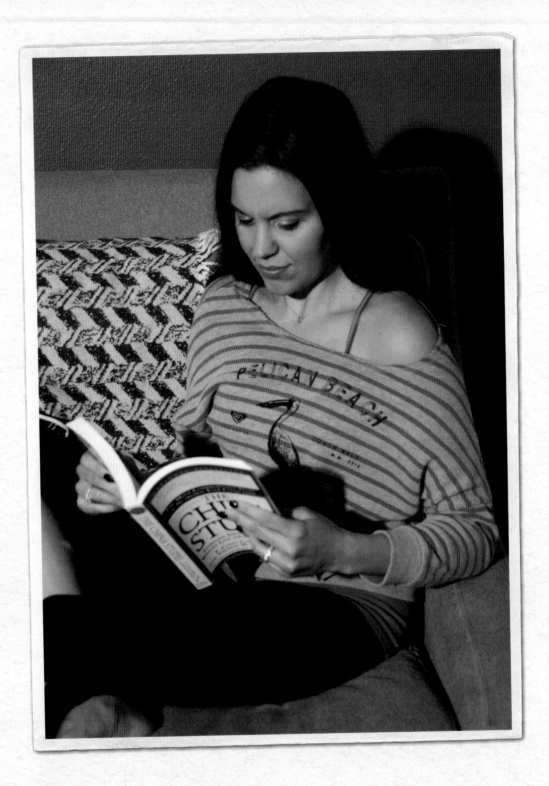

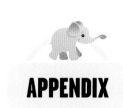

APPENDIX

learn more about plant-based living

This section contains books, films, and online resources
for a variety of plant-based topics.

animal welfare

BOOKS

Eating Animals by Jonathan Safran Foer (Back Bay Books, 2010).
Why We Love Dogs, Eat Pigs, and Wear Cows: An Introduction to Carnism by
Melanie Joy (Conari Press, 2011).

FILMS

Animals Like Us: Business
Blackfish
The Cove
Dolphins: Deep Thinkers
Frankensteer
Mad Cowboy
March of the Penguins
Peaceable Kingdom
Vegucated
We Feed the World
Whale Wars (TV series)

ONLINE RESOURCES

People for the Ethical Treatment of Animals (PETA): http://www.peta.org
Humane Society of the United States: http://www.humanesociety.org
Mercy for Animals: http://www.mercyforanimals.org
PAWS: http://www.paws.org (Happy Herbivore donates a portion of its proceeds
to this charity)
Compassion Over Killing: http://www.cok.net

the environment

BOOKS

Comfortably Unaware: What We Choose to Eat Is Killing Us and Our Planet by Richard A. Oppenlander (Beaufort Books, 2012).

Diet for a New America: How Your Food Choices Affect Your Health, Happiness and the Future of Life on Earth by John Robbins (HJ Kramer/New World Library; 2012, second edition).

Food Choice and Sustainability: Why Buying Local, Eating Less Meat, and Taking Baby Steps Won't Work by Dr. Richard A. Oppenlander (Langdon Street Press, 2013).

The Food Revolution: How Your Diet Can Help Save Your Life and Our World by John Robbins (Conari Press, 2010).

FILMS

Addicted to Plastic

Cowspiracy: The Sustainability Secret

Dive!

Earth (Disney documentary)

Garbage Island

An Inconvenient Truth

Ingredients

King Corn

Mission Blue

More Than Honey

National Geographic: Human Footprint

No Impact Man

SEED: The Untold Story

Tapped

Trashed

Vanishing of the Bees

The Witness

fitness and athletics

BOOKS

The All-Pro Diet: Lose Fat, Build Muscle, and Live Like a Champion by Tony Gonzalez and Mitzi Dulan (Rodale, 2009).

Eat and Run: My Unlikely Journey to Ultramarathon Greatness by Scott Jurek and Steve Friedman (Houghton Mifflin Harcourt, 2013).

The Engine 2 Diet: The Texas Firefighter's 28-Day Save-Your-Life Plan That Lowers Cholesterol and Burns Away the Pounds by Rip Esselstyn (Wellness Central, 2009).

Finding Ultra: Rejecting Middle Age, Becoming One of the World's Fittest Men, and Discovering Myself by Rich Roll (Crown Archetype, 2012).

No Meat Athlete: Run on Plants and Discover Your Fittest, Fastest, Happiest Self by Matt Frazier and Matthew Ruscigno (Fair Winds Press, 2013).

Thrive: The Vegan Nutrition Guide to Optimal Performance in Sports and Life by Brendan Brazier (Da Capo Lifelong Books, 2008).

Thrive Fitness: The Vegan-Based Training Program for Maximum Strength, Health, and Fitness by Brendan Brazier (Da Capo Lifelong Books, 2009).

The Vegan Athlete: Maximizing Your Health and Fitness While Maintaining a Compassionate Lifestyle by Ben Greene and Brett Stewart (Ulysses Press, 2013).

Vegan Bodybuilding & Fitness by Robert Cheeke (Healthy Living Publications, 2010).

Vegetarian Sports Nutrition by D. Enette Larson-Meyer (Human Kinetics, 2007).

FILMS

Strongest Hearts (web series, http://www.strongesthearts.org)

See *Forks Over Knives* in the Health section

ONLINE RESOURCES

"Carl Lewis on Being Vegan," EarthSave.org: http://www.earthsave.org/lifestyle/carllewis.htm

"Eat Better, Perform Better," the Vegetarian Resource Group: http://www.vrg.org/nutshell/athletes.htm

Vegan Bodybuilding & Fitness: http://www.veganbodybuilding.com

Vegan Cycling: http://cycling.davenoisy.com

Vegan Fitness: http://www.veganfitness.net/home

food addiction

BOOKS

Artisan Vegan Cheese by Miyoko Schinner (Book Publishing Company, 2012).

Breaking the Food Seduction: The Hidden Reasons Behind Food Cravings—And 7 Steps to End Them Naturally by Neal D. Barnard and Joanne Stepaniak (St. Martin's Griffin, 2004, reprint edition).

The End of Overeating: Taking Control of the Insatiable American Appetite by David A. Kessler (Rodale Books, 2010, reprint edition).

Mindless Eating: Why We Eat More Than We Think by Brian Wansink (Bantam; 2010, reprint edition).

The Pleasure Trap: Mastering the Hidden Force That Undermines Health & Happiness by Douglas J. Lisle and Alan Goldhamer (Book Publishing Company, 2006).

Salt Sugar Fat: How the Food Giants Hooked Us by Michael Moss (Random House, 2013).

Shrink Yourself: Break Free from Emotional Eating Forever by Roger Gould (Wiley, 2007).

The Ultimate Uncheese Cookbook by Jo Stepaniak (Book Publishing Company, 2003).

FILM

Addicted to Pleasure: Sugar (BBC documentary)

health

BOOKS

21-Day Weight Loss Kickstart: Boost Metabolism, Lower Cholesterol, and Dramatically Improve Your Health by Neal D. Barnard (Hachette Book Group, 2011).

Building Bone Vitality: A Revolutionary Diet Plan to Prevent Bone Loss and Reverse Osteoporosis—Without Dairy Foods, Calcium, Estrogen, or Drugs by Amy Lanou and Michael Castleman (McGraw-Hill, 2009).

The China Study: The Most Comprehensive Study of Nutrition Ever Conducted and the Startling Implications for Diet, Weight Loss and Long-term Health by T. Colin Campbell and Thomas M. Campbell II (BenBella Books, 2006).

Dr. Neal Barnard's Program for Reversing Diabetes: The Scientifically Proven System for Reversing Diabetes without Drugs by Neal D. Barnard (Rodale Books, 2008).

The Engine 2 Diet: The Texas Firefighter's 28-Day Save-Your-Life Plan That Lowers Cholesterol and Burns Away the Pounds by Rip Esselstyn (Wellness Central, 2009).

Food Over Medicine: The Conversation That Could Save Your Life by Pamela A. Popper and Glen Merzer (BenBella Books, 2013).

Forks Over Knives: The Plant-Based Way to Health edited by Gene Stone (The Experiment, 2011).

The Forks Over Knives Plan: How to Transition to the Life-Saving, Whole-Food, Plant-Based Diet by Alona Pulde and Matthew Lederman (Touchstone, 2014).

Healthy at 100: The Scientifically Proven Secrets of the World's Healthiest and Longest-Lived Peoples by John Robbins (Ballantine Books, 2007).

Keep It Simple, Keep It Whole: Your Guide To Optimum Health by Alona Pulde and Matthew Lederman (Exsalus Health & Wellness Center, 2009).

The Low-Carb Fraud by T. Colin Campbell with Howard Jacobson (BenBella Books, 2014).

The McDougall Program for Maximum Weight Loss by John A. McDougall (Plume, 1995).

My Beef with Meat: The Healthiest Argument for Eating a Plant-Strong Diet by Rip Esselstyn (Hachette Book Group, 2013).

The Pillars of Health: Your Foundations for Lifelong Wellness by John Pierre (Hay House, 2013).

Prevent and Reverse Heart Disease: The Revolutionary, Scientifically Proven, Nutrition-Based Cure by Caldwell B. Esselstyn Jr. (Avery Trade, 2008).

The Starch Solution: Eat the Foods You Love, Regain Your Health, and Lose the Weight for Good! by John A. McDougall and Mary McDougall (Rodale Books, 2013).

Whole: Rethinking the Science of Nutrition by T. Colin Campbell with Howard Jacobson (BenBella Books, 2013).

FILMS

The Beautiful Truth
Contagion
A Delicate Balance

Dying to Have Known
Food, Inc.
Forks Over Knives
Frontline: Sick Around America
Got the Facts on Milk?
Happy (documentary)
Killer at Large: Why Obesity is America's Greatest Threat
May I Be Frank
Planeat
Processed People
Super Size Me

for kids

BOOKS

Benji Bean Sprout Doesn't Eat Meat by Sarah Rudy (SK Publishing, 2004).
Charlotte's Web by E. B. White (HarperCollins; reprint edition, 2006).
Cows Are Vegetarian: A Book for Vegetarian Kids by Ann Bradley (Healthways, 1992).
The Giving Tree by Shel Silverstein (HarperCollins, 1964).
Herb, the Vegetarian Dragon by Jules Bass and Debbie Harter (Barefoot Books, 2007).
The Lorax by Dr. Seuss (Random House, 1971).
Madeline and the Bad Hat by Ludwig Bemelmans (Viking Press, 1957).
That's Why We Don't Eat Animals: A Book About Vegans, Vegetarians, and All Living Things by Ruby Roth (North Atlantic Books, 2009).
Yoko by Rosemary Wells (Disney-Hyperion; reprint edition, 2009).

FILMS

Babe
Bears (Disney documentary)
Charlotte's Web (1973, 2006)
Happy Feet
Ratatouille
WALL-E
What's on Your Plate?

ONLINE RESOURCES

"Feeding Vegan Kids," The Vegetarian Resource Group: www.vrg.org/nutshell/
   kids.php

"The Kind Life—Mama," Alicia Silverstone: thekindlife.com/blog/category/mama/

"Nutrition for Kids: A Dietary Approach to Lifelong Health," Physicians
   Committee for Responsible Medicine: support.pcrm.org/site/DocServer/
   Nutrition_for_Kids.pdf?docID=801

"Vegetarian Diets for Children: Right from the Start," Physicians
   Committee for Responsible Medicine: pcrm.org/health/diets/vegdiets/
   vegetarian-diets-for-children-right-from-the-start

meat and masculinity

BOOKS

The Sexual Politics of Meat: A Feminist-Vegetarian Critical Theory by Carol
   Adams (Continuum International Publishing Group, 1990, first edition).

The Heretic's Feast: A History of Vegetarianism by Colin Spencer (University
   Press of New England, 1995).

FILMS

An Emasculating Truth

The Mask You Live In (2015)

Tough Guise: Violence, Media and the Crisis in Masculinity

parenting

BOOKS

The Complete Idiot's Guide to Vegan Eating for Kids by Dana Villamanga and
   Andrew Villamanga (Alpha Books, 2010).

Creating Healthy Children by Karen Ranzi (SHC Publishing, 2010).

Disease-Proof Your Child: Feeding Kids Right by Joel Fuhrman (St. Martin's
   Press, 2006).

Dr. Attwood's Low-Fat Prescription Diet for Kids by Charles Attwood (Penguin
   Books, 1996).

Healthy Eating for Life for Children by the Physicians Committee for Responsible
   Medicine (Wiley, 2002).
Raising Vegetarian Children: A Guide to Good Health and Family Harmony by
   Joanne Stepaniak and Vesanto Melina (McGraw-Hill, 2002).
Raising Vegan Children in a Non-Vegan World: A Complete Guide for Parents by
   Erin Pavlina (VegFamily, 2003).

FILMS

Babies
Frontline: The Medicated Child
My Toxic Baby

ONLINE RESOURCES

The Kind Life: thekindlife.com
Physicians Committe for Responsible Medicine: http://www.pcrm.org/

pregnancy

BOOKS

*The Everything Vegan Pregnancy Book: All You Need to Know for a Healthy
   Pregnancy That Fits Your Lifestyle* by Reed Mangels (Adams Media, 2011).
*The Kind Mama: A Simple Guide to Supercharged Fertility, a Radiant Pregnancy,
   a Sweeter Birth, and a Healthy, More Beautiful Beginning* by Alicia Silverstone
   (Rodale, 2014).
*Skinny Bitch Bun in the Oven: A Gutsy Guide to Becoming One Hot (and Healthy)
   Mother!* by Rory Freedman and Kim Barnouin (Running Press, 2008).
Vegan Pregnancy Survival Guide by Sayward Rebhal (Herbivore Books, 2011).
Your Vegetarian Pregnancy: A Month-to-Month Guide to Health and Nutrition by
   Holly Roberts (Simon & Schuster, 2003).

FILMS

The Business of Being Born
More Business of Being Born
Pregnant in America

ONLINE RESOURCES

"Pregnancy," The Vegan Society: http://www.vegansociety.com/resources/
nutrition-health/eating-well-early-life

"Pregnancy and the Vegan Diet," Vegetarian Resource Group:
www.vrg.org/nutrition/veganpregnancy.php

"Vegetarian Diets for Pregnancy," Physicians Committee for Responsible
Medicine: pcrm.org/health/diets/vegdiets/vegetarian-diets-for-pregnancy

religion and politics

BOOKS

Salt Sugar Fat: How the Food Giants Hooked Us by Michael Moss (Random
House, 2013).

FILMS

The Corporation

Eating Mercifully: Christian Perspectives on Factory Farming

Fast Food Nation (film)

The Harvest/La Cosecha

Hot Coffee

Jiro Dreams of Sushi

A Place at the Table

A Sacred Duty: Applying Jewish Values to Help Heal the World

Sicko

Who Killed the Electric Car?

notes

chapter 1

1. Douglas J. Lisle and Alan Goldhamer, *The Pleasure Trap* (Summertown, TN: Book Publishing Company, 2006).

2. D. Feskanich et al., "Milk, Dietary Calcium, and Bone Fractures in Women: A 12-Year Prospective Study," *American Journal of Public Health* 87, no. 6 (June 1997): 992–97.

3. "When Friends Ask: 'Why Don't You Drink Milk?'," *The McDougall Newsletter* 6, no. 3 (March 2007), http://www.drmcdougall.com/misc/2007nl/mar/dairy.htm.

4. "Lactose Intolerance: Information for Health Care Providers," January 2006, U.S. Department of Health and Human Services, National Institutes of Health, https://www.nichd.nih.gov/publications/pubs/documents/NICHD_MM_Lactose_FS_rev.pdf.

5. S. J. Moschos and C. S. Mantzoros, "The Role of the IGF System in Cancer: From Basic to Clinical Studies and Clinical Applications," *Oncology* 63, no. 4 (November 2002): 317–32.

6. T. Colin Campbell with Howard Jacobson, *Whole: Rethinking the Science of Nutrition* (Dallas: BenBella Books, 2013).

7. "The Protein Myth," Physicians Committee for Responsible Medicine, accessed September 16, 2014, www.pcrm.org/health/diets/vegdiets/how-can-i-get-enough-protein-the-protein-myth.

8. Jeff Novick, "The Myth of Complementary Protein," Forks Over Knives (blog), June 3, 2013, http://www.forksoverknives.com/the-myth-of-complementary-protein.

9. Ibid.

10. R. Rozenek et al., "Effects of high-calorie supplements on body composition and muscular strength following resistance training," *Journal of Sports Medicine and Physical Fitness* (September 2002): 340-47.

11. Ibid.

12. "Organic Meats Are Not Health Foods," Physicians Committee for Responsible Medicine, accessed September 16, 2014, www.pcrm.org/health/health-topics/organic-meats-are-not-health-foods.

13. T. Colin Campbell, "Dr. Campbell Responds to Dr. Mercola," VegSource, September 11, 2009, http://www.vegsource.com/news/2009/09/dr-campbell-responds-to-dr-mercola.html.

14. R. Sharpe and N. Skakkebaek, "Are Oestrogens Involved in Falling Sperm Counts and Disorders of the Male Reproductive Tract?," *Lancet* 341, no. 8857 (May 1993): 1392–95.

15. "FAQ: Why Does the Diet Eliminate Oil Entirely?," Dr. Esselstyn's Prevent & Reverse Heart Disease Program, accessed September 16, 2014, http://www.dresselstyn.com/site/faq.

16. "When Friends Ask: 'Why Do You Avoid Adding Vegetable Oils?'," *The McDougall Newsletter* 6, no. 8 (August 2007), http://drmcdougall.com/misc/2007nl/aug/oils.htm.

17. "FAQ."

18. "Omega-3 Fatty Acids," The World's Healthiest Foods, George Mateljan Foundation, accessed September 16, 2014, http://www.whfoods.com/genpage.php?tname=nutrient&dbid=84.

19. The Mediterranean diet focuses on eating primarily fruits, vegetables, olive oil, grains, legumes, nuts, and seeds at every meal, plus fish or seafood twice a week. Dairy, eggs, meats, and sweets are eaten less often.

20. Rip Esselstyn, *My Beef with Meat: The Healthiest Argument for Eating a Plant-Strong Diet* (New York: Hachette Book Group, 2013), 15.

21. "World's Fattest Countries," *Forbes*, February 8, 2007, http://www.forbes.com/2007/02/07/worlds-fattest-countries-forbeslife-cx_ls_0208worldfat.html.

22. Vitamin D is made in the body as the result of exposure to sunlight. For most people, five to fifteen minutes of sun a day between the hours of 10 a.m. and 3 p.m., exposing the arms and legs, or the hands, face, and arms, during the spring, summer, and fall, is sufficient. However, individuals who live in cold or overcast climates, or otherwise have inadequate exposure to sunlight, regardless of their diet, should talk to their doctor about taking a supplement.

23. Esselstyn, *My Beef with Meat*, 19–21.

24. Esselstyn, *My Beef with Meat*.

25. All values are taken from their listings on The World's Healthiest Foods website, The George Mateljan Foundation, http://www.whfoods.com.

chapter 2

1. "Lifetime Risk of Developing or Dying from Cancer," American Cancer Society, last modified September 5, 2013, www.cancer.org/cancer/cancerbasics/lifetime-probability-of-developing-or-dying-from-cancer.

2. Caldwell B. Esselstyn, Jr., *Prevent and Reverse Heart Disease: The Revolutionary, Scientifically Proven Nutrition-Based Cure* (Avery Trade, 2008).

3. Mark Hyman, "The One Diet That Can Cure Most Disease: Part I," DrHyman.com (blog), July 3, 2013, http://drhyman.com/blog/2013/05/17/the-one-diet-that-can-cure-most-disease-part-i/#close.

4. As discussed in *Forks Over Knives*, directed by Lee Fulkerson (Monica Beach Media, 2011).

5. T. Colin Campbell and Thomas M. Campbell II, *The China Study: The Most Comprehensive Study of Nutrition Ever Conducted and the Startling Implications for Diet, Weight Loss and Long-term Health* (Dallas: BenBella Books, 2006).

6. Neal Barnard, "Chocolate, Cheese, Meat, and Sugar—Physically Addictive," www.youtube.com/watch?v=5VWi6dXCT7I.

7. Lisle and Goldhamer, *The Pleasure Trap.*

8. "Allergy Facts," American College of Allergy, Asthma & Immunology, accessed September 16, 2014, http://www.acaai.org/allergist/news/Pages/Allergy_Facts.aspx.

9. "Leukotrienes & Lipoxins," St. Edward's University Department of Chemistry & Biochemistry, accessed September 16, 2014, http://www.cs.stedwards.edu/chem/Chemistry/CHEM43/CHEM43/Leukotr/REGCNTRL.HTML.

10. Neal D. Barnard, "Ask the Doc: How Can I Stop Seasonal Sniffles?," *Vegetarian Times*, accessed September 16, 2014, http://www.vegetariantimes.com/article/ask-the-doc-seasonal-allergies.

11. M. Kimata et al., "Effects of Luteolin, Quercetin and Baicalein on Immunoglobulin E-mediated Mediator Release from Human Cultured Mast Cells," *Clinical & Experimental Allergy* 30, no. 4 (2000): 501–8, http://www.ncbi.nlm.nih.gov/pubmed/10718847.

12. M. Czarnecka-Operacz et al., "Oral allergy syndrome in patients with airborne pollen allergy treated with specific immunotherapy," *Acta Dermatovenerologica Croatica* 2008;16(1):19-24, http://www.ncbi.nlm.nih.gov/pubmed/18358104.

13. "Asthma in the US," U.S. Centers for Disease Control and Prevention, last modified May 3, 2011, http://www.cdc.gov/vitalsigns/asthma; U.S. National Heart, Lung, and Blood Institute, "What Is Asthma?," last modified August 4, 2014, http://www.nhlbi.nih.gov/health/health-topics/topics/asthma.

14. "Asthma: Nutritional Considerations," NutritionMD, accessed September 16, 2014, http://www.nutritionmd.org/health_care_providers/respiratory/asthma_nutrition.html.

15. "Better Breathing from Diet," *The McDougall Newsletter* 9, no. 5 (May 2010), https://www.drmcdougall.com/misc/2010nl/may/breathing.htm.

16. Deanna Ferrerri, "Childhood Diet Linked to Asthma Prevalence, Adult Diet Linked to Asthma Severity," Dr. Fuhrman's Disease Proof (blog), September 27, 2010, http://www.diseaseproof.com/archives/asthma-childhood-diet-linked-to-asthma-prevalence-adult-diet-linked-to-asthma-severity.html.

17. "Asthma in the US."

18. "Asthma: Nutritional Considerations."

19. Ferreri, "Childhood Diet."

20. Heiner Boeing et al., "Critical review: vegetables and fruit in the prevention of chronic diseases," *European Journal of Nutrition* 51, no. 1 (2012): 637–63, http://www.ncbi.nlm.nih.gov/pmc/articles/PMC3419346.

21. "Asthma: Nutritional Considerations."

22. Ibid.

23. Ibid.

24. O. Lindahl et al., "Vegan Regimen with Reduced Medication in the Treatment of Bronchial Asthma," *Journal of Asthma* 22, no. 1 (1985): 45–55, http://www.ncbi.nlm.nih.gov/pubmed/4019393.

25. Ferreri, "Childhood Diet."

26. "Allergic Reactions to Food," Dr. McDougall's Health & Medical Center, accessed September 16, 2014, https://www.drmcdougall.com/health/education/health-science/common-health-problems/allergic-reactions-to-food.

27. Benjamin Caballero, "The Global Epidemic of Obesity: An Overview," *Epidemiologic Reviews* 29, no. 1 (2007): 1–5, http://epirev.oxfordjournals.org/content/29/1/1.long.

28. Andrew Pollack, "A.M.A. Recognizes Obesity as a Disease," *New York Times*, June 18, 2013, http://www.nytimes.com/2013/06/19/business/ama-recognizes-obesity-as-a-disease.html.

29. "Controlling the Global Obesity Epidemic," World Health Organization, accessed September 16, 2014, http://www.who.int/nutrition/topics/obesity/en.

30. "FastStats: Obesity and Overweight," U.S. Centers for Disease Control and Prevention, last modified May 14, 2013, http://www.cdc.gov/nchs/fastats/obesity-overweight.htm.

31. "Obesity among Children Increases," Physicians Committee for Responsible Medicine, April 9, 2014, http://www.pcrm.org/health/medNews/obesity-among-children-increases.

32. E. Jequier and G. A. Bray, "Low-Fat Diets Are Preferred," *American Journal of Medicine* 113, suppl. 9B (2002): 41S–46S.

33. Sara N. Bleich, David Cutler, Christopher Murray, and Alyce Adams, "Why Is the Developed World Obese?," *Annual Review of Public Health* 29 (2008): 273–95, http://www.annualreviews.org/doi/abs/10.1146/annurev.publhealth.29.020907.090954.

34. J. P. Adams and P. G. Murphy, "Obesity in Anaesthesia and Intensive Care," *British Journal of Anaesthesia* 85 (2000): 91–108, http://bja.oxfordjournals.org/content/85/1/91.full.

35. Neal D. Barnard, "Cheese and Obesity," Dr. Barnard's Blog, Physicians Committee for Responsible Medicine, January 24, 2012, http://www.pcrm.org/media/blog/jan2012/cheese-and-obesity.

36. Ibid.

37. Ibid.

38. "Obesity," Dr. McDougall's Health & Medical Center, accessed September 16, 2014, https://www.drmcdougall.com/health/education/health-science/common-health-problems/obesity.

39. "Obesity: Nutritional Considerations," NutritionMD, accessed September 16, 2014, http://www.nutritionmd.org/health_care_providers/general_nutrition/obesity_nutrition.html.

40. M. F. McCarty, "The Origins of Western Obesity: A Role for Animal Protein?," *Medical Hypotheses* 54, no. 3 (2000): 488–94, http://www.ncbi.nlm.nih.gov/pubmed/10783494.

41. "Obesity: Nutritional Considerations."

42. Ibid.

43. "New DIETs: New Dietary Interventions Enhancing the Treatment for Weight Loss," ClinicalTrials.gov, U.S. National Institutes of Health, accessed September 16, 2014, http://clinicaltrials.gov/show/NCT01742572.

44. "Plant-Based Diets Show More Weight Loss Without Emphasizing Caloric Restriction," Obesity.org, accessed January 2015, http://www.obesity.org/news-center/plant-based-diets-show-more-weight-loss-without-emphasizing-caloric-restriction.htm.

45. N. D. Barnard et al. "The Effects of a Low-Fat, Plant-Based Dietary Intervention on Body Weight, Metabolism, and Insulin Sensitivity," *American Journal of Medicine* 118 (2005): 991–97.

46. "Obesity: Nutritional Considerations."

47. Michael Greger, "Thousands of Vegans Studied," NutritionFacts.org video, 3:31, February 26, 2011, http://nutritionfacts.org/video/thousands-of-vegans-studied.

48. United Nations Environmental Programme, International Panel for Sustainable Resource Management, Assessing the Environmental Impacts of Consumption and Production: Priority Products and Materials, A Report of the Working Group on the Environmental Impacts of Products and Materials to the International Panel for Sustainable Resource Management (Paris: United Nations Environmental Programme, 2010), www.unep.org/resourcepanel/Publications/PriorityProducts/tabid/56053/Default.aspx.

49. World Health Organization, Department of Nutrition for Health and Development, Turning the Tide of Malnutrition: Responding to the Challenge of the 21st Century (Geneva: World Health Organization, 2000), http://whqlibdoc.who.int/hq/2000/WHO_NHD_00.7.pdf.

50. Richard A. Oppenlander, *Comfortably Unaware: Global Depletion and Food Responsibility . . . What You Choose to Eat Is Killing Our Planet* (Minneapolis: Langdon Street Press, 2011).

51. "U.S. Could Feed 800 Million People with Grain That Livestock Eat, Cornell Ecologist Advises Animal Scientists," *Cornell Chronicle*, last modified August 7, 1997, http://www.news.cornell.edu/stories/1997/08/us-could-feed-800-million-people-grain-livestock-eat.

52. John Robbins, *Diet for a New America* (Walpole, NH: Stillpoint, 1987), 353.

53. "U.S. Could Feed 800 Million People."

54. Marcia Kreith, *Water Inputs in California Food Production* (Sacramento: Water Education Foundation, 1991), http://www.sakia.org/cms/fileadmin/content/irrig/general/kreith_1991_water_inputs_in_ca_food_production-excerpt.pdf.

55. "Meat Production Wastes Natural Resources," People for the Ethical Treatment of Animals, accessed March 31, 2014, http://www.peta.org/issues/animals-used-for-food/meat-wastes-natural-resources.

56. "Public-Supply Water Use," U.S. Geological Survey, accessed March 31, 2014, http://water.usgs.gov/edu/wups.html.

57. Tom Gleeson et al., "Water Balance of Global Aquifers Revealed by Groundwater Footprint," *Nature* 488 (2012): 197–200, http://www.nature.com/nature/journal/v488/n7410/full/nature11295.html.

58. "U.S. Could Feed 800 Million People."

59. Ibid.

60. Esselstyn, *My Beef with Meat*, 77.

61. "U.S. Could Feed 800 Million People."

62. "Facts about Pollution from Livestock Farms," National Resources Defense Council, last modified February 21, 2013, http://www.nrdc.org/water/pollution/ffarms.asp.

63. Susan W. Gay and Katharine F. Knowlton, "Ammonia Emissions and Animal Agriculture," Virginia Cooperative Extension, last modified May 1, 2009, http://pubs.ext.vt.edu/442/442-110/442-110.html.

64. Fred Pearce, "Methane: The Hidden Greenhouse Gas," *New Scientist* (May 6, 1989), http://www.newscientist.com/article/mg12216635.100-methane-the-hidden-greenhouse-gas.html.

65. "Rainforests: Facts about Rainforests," The Nature Conservancy, accessed March 31, 2014, www.nature.org/ourinitiatives/urgentissues/rainforests/rainforests-facts.xml.

66. John Robbins, *The Food Revolution: How Your Diet Can Help Save Your Life and Our World* (San Francisco: Conari Press, 2010), 256.

67. Esselstyn, *My Beef with Meat*, 78.

68. "IV. Worker Health and Safety in the Meat and Poultry Industry," *Blood, Sweat, and Fear*, Human Rights Watch (New York: 2004), 24.

69. "Slaughterhouse Workers," Food Empowerment Project, accessed September 17, 2014, http://www.foodispower.org/slaughterhouse-workers.

70. Sameer Farooq, "Exploitation in the 21st Century: Illegal Immigrants in the Meatpacking Industry," BU Arts & Sciences Writing Program, accessed September 17, 2014, http://www.bu.edu/writingprogram/journal/past-issues/issue-4/farooq.

71. "Factory Farm Workers," Food Empowerment Project, accessed September 17, 2014, http://www.foodispower.org/factory-farm-workers.

72. Steven Greenhouse, "No Days Off at Foie Gras Farm; Workers Complain, but Owner Cites Stress on Ducks," *New York Times*, April 2, 2001, http://www.nytimes.com/2001/04/02/nyregion/no-days-off-at-foie-gras-farm-workers-complain-but-owner-cites-stress-on-ducks.html.

73. "Factory Farm Workers."

chapter 3

1. "The McDougall Diet for Pregnancy," The McDougall Newsletter 10, no. 1 (January 2011), https://www.drmcdougall.com/misc/2011nl/jan/pregnancy.htm.

2. National Research Council, Dietary Reference Intakes for Energy, Carbohydrate, Fiber, Fat, Fatty Acids, Cholesterol, Protein, and Amino Acids (Washington, DC: The National Academies Press, 2005).

3. National Research Council, Dietary Reference Intakes for Calcium, Phosphorus, Magnesium, Vitamin D, and Fluoride (Washington, DC: The National Academies Press, 1997).

4. "Vegetarian Diets for Pregnancy," Physicians Committee for Responsible Medicine, accessed September 17, 2014, http://www.pcrm.org/health/diets/vegdiets/vegetarian-diets-for-pregnancy.

5. Ibid.

6. "Iron and Iron Deficiency," U.S. Centers for Disease Control and Prevention, last modified February 23, 2011, http://www.cdc.gov/nutrition/everyone/basics/vitamins/iron.html.

7. "Folate: Dietary Supplement Fact Sheet," U.S. National Institutes of Health, last modified December 14, 2012, http://ods.od.nih.gov/factsheets/Folate-HealthProfessional.

8. Ibid.

9. "Vitamin B$_{12}$ Deficiency—The Meat-Eaters' Last Stand," *The McDougall Newsletter* 6, no. 11 (November 2007), http://drmcdougall.com/misc/2007nl/nov/b12.htm.

10. "Vegetarian Diets for Pregnancy."

11. K. Marsh and J. Brand-Miller, "The Optimal Diet for Women with Polycystic Ovary Syndrome?" *British Journal of Nutrition* 94, no. 2 (August 2005): 154–65.

12. "Diet Cured My Endometriosis and Helped Me Have My Son," Dr. McDougall's Health & Medical Center, accessed September 17, 2014, http://www.drmcdougall.com/stars/051205starpaula.html.

13. Øjvind Lindegaard et al., "Thrombotic Stroke and Myocardial Infarction with Hormonal Contraception," *New England Journal of Medicine* 366 (June 2012): 2257–66, http://www.nejm.org/doi/full/10.1056/NEJMoa1111840.

14. "Hormone Dependent Diseases (Male & Female)," Dr. McDougall's Health & Medical Center, accessedSeptember 17, 2014, http://www.drmcdougall.com/health/education/health-science/common-health-problems/hormone-dependent-diseases-male-female/.

15. "Diet Cured My Endometriosis."

16. "Hormone Dependent Diseases (Male & Female)."

17. "A Natural Approach to Menopause," Physicians Committee for Responsible Medicine, accessed September 17, 2014, http://www.pcrm.org/health/health-topics/a-natural-approach-to-menopause.

18. Ibid.

19. Paul Rozin et al., "Is Meat Male? A Quantitative Multi-Method Framework to Establish Metaphoric Relationships," *Journal of Consumer Research* 39, no. 3 (October 2012): 629–43.

20. "A Pant-Strong PSA," Engine 2 Diet (blog), March 6, 2012, http://engine2diet.com/the-daily-beet/a-pant-strong-psa.

21. Lindsay S. Nixon, "Meet Our Plant-Based (Vegan) Guys: A Look at Men's Perspective & Experience (Part 1)," Happy Herbivore (blog), June 11, 2013, http://happyherbivore.com/2013/06/plant-based-vegan-men-part-1.

22. "Raise the Flag with a Vegan Diet," YouTube video, 3:49, posted by "Forks Over Knives," January 23, 2012, https://www.youtube.com/watch?v=z4ECnqXQpDA.

23. "Meat Consumption and Cancer Risk," Physicians Committee for Responsible Medicine, accessed September 17, 2014, www.pcrm.org/health/cancer-resources/diet-cancer/facts/meat-consumption-and-cancer-risk.

24. "FAQ: Prostate Cancer—Does Plant Based Eating Help Prostate Cancer?" Dr. Esselstyn's Prevent & Reverse Heart Disease Program, accessed September 16, 2014, http://www.dresselstyn.com/site/faq.

25. "Hormone Dependent Diseases (Male & Female)."

26. Ibid.

27. If your school is peanut-free, try almond butter. If your school is completely nut-free, try sunflower seed butter. A popular/common brand is SunButter (sold at Walmart and most supermarkets).

chapter 4

1. Pamela A. Popper, *Food Over Medicine: The Conversation That Could Save Your Life* (Dallas: BenBella Books, 2013), 13.

2. Campbell and Jacobson, *Whole*, 65.

chapter 6

1. "Chocolate, Cheese, Meat, and Sugar: Physically Addictive," YouTube video, 40:12, posted by "VegSource," January 20, 2010, http://www.youtube.com/watch?v=5VWi6dXCT7I.

2. T. Colin Campbell and Thomas M. Campbell II, *The China Study: The Most Comprehensive Study of Nutrition Ever Conducted and the Startling Implications for Diet, Weight Loss and Long-term Health* (Dallas: BenBella Books, 2006).

3. Tara Parker-Pope, "How the Food Makers Captured Our Brains," *New York Times*, June 22, 2009, http://www.nytimes.com/2009/06/23/health/23well.html.

4. Lisle and Goldhamer, *The Pleasure Trap.*

5. Deepak Chopra, *The Seven Spiritual Laws of Success* (San Rafael, CA: Amber-Allen 1994).

6. Ibid.

7. Academy of Achievement, "Johnny Cash: Interview," June 25, 1993, last modified December 6, 2013, http://www.achievement.org/autodoc/page/cas0int-1.

8. "Alcohol Consumption," Dr. McDougall's Health & Medical Center, accessed September 17, 2014, http://www.drmcdougall.com/alcohol.html.

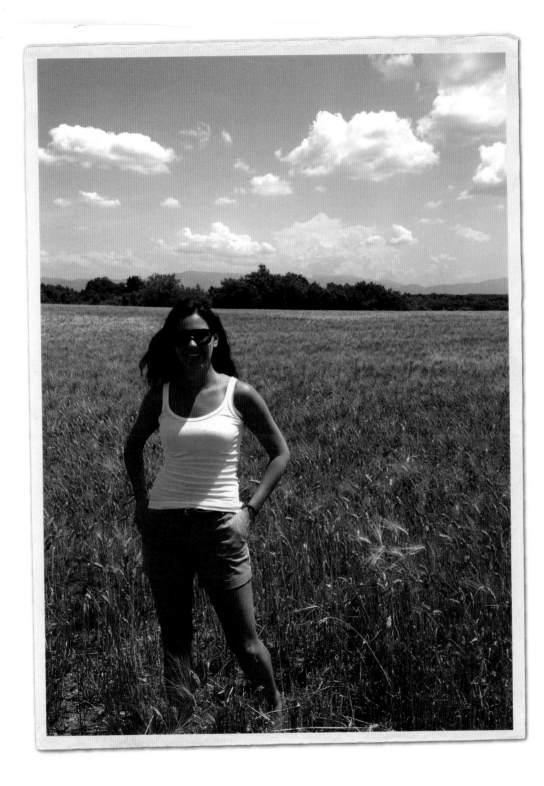

about the author

Lindsay S. Nixon is the bestselling author of the Happy Herbivore cookbook series: *The Happy Herbivore Cookbook* (2011), *Everyday Happy Herbivore* (2011), *Happy Herbivore Abroad* (2012), *Happy Herbivore Light & Lean* (2013), *The Happy Herbivore Guide to Plant-Based Living* (2014, e-book only), and now *Happy Herbivore Holidays & Gatherings.* Nixon has sold over 200,000 copies of her cookbooks.

Nixon has been featured on the Food Network and *The Dr. Oz Show*, and she has spoken at Google's Pittsburgh office about health, plant-based food, and her success. She is also a teaching professor at the Center for Nutrition Studies at eCornell and her recipes have been featured in the *New York Times*, *Vegetarian Times* magazine, *Shape* magazine, *Bust*, *Women's Health*, WebMD, and numerous other publications. Nixon's work has also been praised and endorsed by notable leaders in the field of nutrition, including Dr. T. Colin Campbell, Dr. Caldwell B. Esselstyn Jr., Dr. Neal Barnard, Dr. John McDougall, and Dr. Pam Popper.

A rising star in the culinary world, Nixon is recognized for her ability to use everyday ingredients to create healthy, low-fat recipes that taste just as delicious as they are nutritious. Learn more about Nixon and try some of her recipes on her award-winning blog, happyherbivore.com. You can also try her 7-Day Meal Plans at getmealplans.com.

Other cookbooks
by Lindsay S. Nixon,
brought to you by BenBella Books

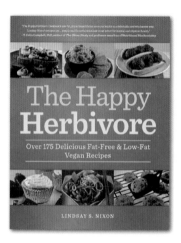

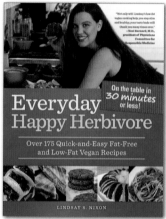

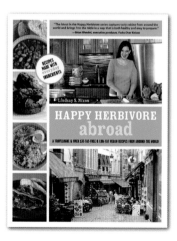

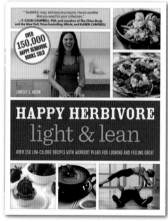

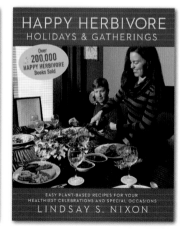

recipe index

AJ's Vegan Parmesan, 239
Banana Boats, 148
Bean Soup, 222
Beef and Broccoli, 221
Belize Bean Quesadillas, 224–225
Butternut and Pea Curry, 226
Caribbean Ragout, 227
"Cheater" Tofu Lettuce Wraps, 228
Creamy Cajun Mustard, 242
Everyday Mushroom Gravy, 243
Golden Dressing, 241
"Honey" Mustard, 245
Indian Lentils & Cabbage, 229
Ketchup, 244
Lemon Takeout Chickpeas, 230

Lime Crème, 242
Mexican Quinoa, 231
Moroccan Carrot Soup, 232
Moroccan Chickpeas, 233
Mushroom & Potato Soup, 234
No-Beef Broth, 195, 238
No-Chicken Broth, 195, 238
Pozole, 235
Quick Queso Sauce, 245
S'mores, 148
Southwestern Loaf, 236
Vegan Mayo, 239
Vegan Sour Cream, 242
Vegan Worcestershire Sauce, 240

subject index

a

Aaron (testimonial), 138–139
acid reflux, 41
acne, 25
adapting recipes, 194–195, 199–200.
    see also substitutions
agar agar, 195
agave/agave nectar, 195, 204

airline/airport foods, 140
ALA (alpha-linolenic acid), 32, 73
alcohol, weight and, 210
allergies
    and diet, 41
    food, 46–50, 196–199
    seasonal, 43–45
almond meal, 198

alternatives. *see* substitutions

Alzheimer's, 42

Ami (testimonial), 158–159

amino acids, 26–27

anecdotal evidence, combating, 178–179

anemia, 25

animal agriculture, 55–57, 60, 62

animal welfare, 61–62, 248

arthritis, 41

asthma, 43–46

athletes, 27, 94–95

athletics resources, 250

attention deficit disorder, 41–42

attitude, 66–67

Aubrey (testimonial), 92–93

autoimmune diseases, 41, 42

avoiding temptation, 174–175

b

backpacking, 146–148

bacon, 178, 179

bacon substitutes, 195

baking

   alternatives for food allergies, 196–199

   plant-based, 199–205

   shopping list for, 218

   substitutions and adaptations in, 194–195

barrier contraceptives, 79

beans, 23, 108

   alternatives to, 197–198

   canned, 109

   as fast food, 118

   and flatulence, 68

   in minimalist meals, 127–129

   as nut substitutes, 197

   during pregnancy, 74

   protein in, 26

   in transition meals, 107

   in travel emergency kit, 149

beef, 57, 195

benefits of plant-based diet, 39–62

   global, 55–62

health benefits, 40–55

Beth (testimonial), 86–77

blood pressure, 28, 29, 51, 59, 77, 88, 138

bodily functions, 68–70

bone loss, 81

breads, 74, 215. *see also* baking

bread substitutes, 120–121

breast-feeding, nutrition during, 71–75

Brian (testimonial), 84–85

broth substitutes, 120

brown rice, 108, 128, 198

brussels sprouts, 68

bulk buying, 116

butter, 178, 179. *see also* dairy foods

buttermilk, 195

butter substitutes, 195, 199, 201

c

calcium, 24, 73, 81

calories, 154–155, 211

Cam, 82, 94, 100 (testimonial)

Campbell, T. Colin, 19, 30, 42

camping, 146–148

cancer, 25, 30, 40–42, 51, 74, 75, 80, 82, 83, 85, 119, 130

candy, vegan, 126

canker sores, 47

canned goods, 121, 128, 215

carob, 205

casein, 154, 155

cashew cream, 157, 195

casomorphins, 154

catered events, 169

cereals, 86, 149

challenges of plant-based lifestyle, 153–179

   avoiding temptation, 174–175

   being "selfish," 175

   combating anecdotal evidence, 178–179

   food addictions, 154–161

   mixed households, 175–178

   negativity, 162, 165–166

   social situations, 167–173

cheese, 52. *see also* dairy foods
  addiction to, 154
  breaking addiction to, 158-159
  plant-based substitutes for, 195
  substitutes for, 157
  vegan substitutes for, 124
chicken substitutes, 195
chickpea miso, 196. 220
children, 86-91
  asthma in, 45
  changes with plant-based lifestyle, 88-89
  drinks, 91
  fats for, 32
  kids' parties, 170
  obesity among, 51
  resources for, 253-254
  school lunches, 90
  snacks, 91
The China Study, 42
chocolate, 205. 210
chocolate chips, 205
Chopra, Deepak, 165. 167
Chris (testimonial), 37
chronic disease, 40-42
cocoa, 204
coconut aminos, 196. 198. 220
coconut milk, 107. 108. 195. 205. 210
coconut oil, 31
coffee, 69. 210
commercial substitutes
  for eggs, 200
  plant-based, 120-122
  for soy, 196-197
  vegan (not plant-based), 122-126
commitment, making, 109. 214
"complete" protein myth, 26-27
condiments
  commercial substitutes for, 121. 125
  shopping list for, 215
conformity, 166
constipation, 25. 47. 69
contraception, 78-80
convenience foods, 109. 116. 210

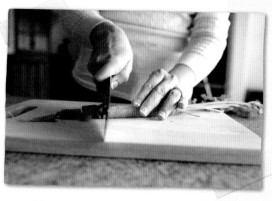

cooking
  alternatives for food allergies, 196-199
  plant-based baking, 199-205
  substitutions and adaptations in
    recipes, 194-195
  time involved in, 117-118
corn alternatives, 198
cost of plant-based diet, 111-112. 116-117
Courtney, 47-49
cravings, 155-156. 160-161
creamers, nondairy, 124
cream substitutes, 195. *see also* dairy foods

d

dairy foods
  addiction to, 154
  as allergens, 196
  and asthma, 46
  breaking addiction to, 157
  eliminating, 103
  plant-based substitutes for, 195
  substitutes for, 157
dairy myth, 24-25
Danzig, Mac, 94
David (testimonial), 28-29. 82
declining food, 170-173
depression, 41. 47
DHA (docosahexaenoic acid), 32. 73
diabetes, 25. 32. 40-42. 51. 55. 82. 108
diarrhea, 47
dieting, 19. 20. 214
dinner invitations, 168-169

disease(s), 118
  and choices of foods, 190
  chronic, 40–42
  obesity as, 51
"don't worry about me" approach, 167–168
dorms, cooking in, 146
Drayton, William, 57
dressing(s)
  shopping list for, 215
  substitutes for, 125, 137

e

ear infections, 25
eating disorders, 163–164
eating out, 132–136
  finding options when, 133–134, 136–137
  veg-friendly cuisines, 134–136
  and weight, 210
eczema, 25, 41, 46, 88, 206
eggs, 46, 103, 196, 199
eggs substitutes, 195, 200–201
elimination, 69
elimination diet, 50, 71
Elondra (testimonial), 63–64
emotional aspect of food, 112, 114–115, 161
endometriosis, 75
energy density, 53–55
environment, 56–57, 60–61
  fossil fuels, 57
  resources about, 249
  water resources, 56–57
EPA (eicosapentaenoic acid), 32, 73
erectile dysfunction, 83
Esselstyn, Caldwell B., Jr., 31, 32, 41, 42
Esselstyn, Rip, 26, 82, 94, 164
essential fatty acids, 73
ethnic markets, 116

f

failure to thrive, 209–211
family, convincing. see leading by example

fast-food restaurants, 134
fatigue, 41, 46, 211
fats. see also oils
  addiction to, 154–155
  breaking addiction to, 157, 160
  as "magic food," 52
  myths about, 31–32
  and obesity, 51–53
fat substitutes, 201
fatty acids, 32, 73
fertility, 75–78
fish oil myth, 32
fish substitutes, 195
fitness resources, 250
flatulence, 68–69
flours, 198
  in baking, 199
  energy density of, 53
  gluten-free, 203
  and weight, 210
  whole-wheat, 202–203
foil-pack cooking, 147
folate, 74
folic acid, 74
food addictions, 117, 154–161
  breaking, 102–103, 155–160
  and changes to taste buds, 161–162
  and cravings, 160–161
  resources on, 251
food allergies/sensitivities, 46–50, 69, 196–199
food pyramid, plant-based, 36
food safety, 147
fossil fuels, 57
freeze-dried meals, 147
friends, convincing. see leading by example
frozen dinner substitutes, 125
frozen foods shopping list, 217
fruits, 23, 108. see also plant-based diet
  and asthma, 46
  cottonseed polish on, 48
  dried, weight and, 210
  energy density of, 53

grilled, 148
  in minimalist meals, 128
  as sugar substitute, 156
  in travel emergency kit, 149
  for traveling, 147
fruit stands, 144
Fuhrman, Joel, 46

g

gas-causing foods, 68–69
gas station foods, 140, 145
gelatin substitutes, 195
generic brands, 116
Gina (testimonial), 206–207
global impact of plant-based diet, 55–62
  environmental factors, 60–61
  fossil fuels, 57
  human and animal welfare, 61–62
  water resources, 56–57
  world hunger, 56
gluten, 196
gluten alternatives, 198
gluten-free baking, 203
gluten-free shopping list, 218
Goldhamer, Alan, 23, 162
"good fat" myth, 31–32
grains, 108

gluten-free, 198
grass-fed myth, 27, 30
grief, stages of, 113
grilled dishes, 136, 137, 146, 148
guests, feeding, 189

h

ham substitutes, 195
Hancock, Herbie, 153
Hayes, Frederick, 168
headaches, 47
health
  and contraceptive use, 79
  resources on, 251–253
  WHO definition of, 40
health benefits of plant-based diet,
  40–55. see also nutrition
  asthma, 43, 45–46
  chronic disease, 40–42
  hidden food allergies/sensitivities, 46–50
  obesity and weight loss, 50–55
  seasonal allergies, 43–45
health food stores, 116
heartburn, 25
heart disease, 25, 32, 40–42, 51, 79, 82, 83,
  97, 104–105, 108
Herbies
  Aaron, 138–139
  Ami, 158–159
  Aubrey, 92 –93
  Beth, 86–77
  Brian, 84–85
  Cam, 100
  Chris, 37
  David, 28–29, 82
  Elondra, 63–64
  Gina, 206–207
  Jeremy, 184–186
  Kim, 190–192
  Michelle (changes in kids), 88–89
  Michelle (eating disorder), 163–164
  Robin, 114–115, 130

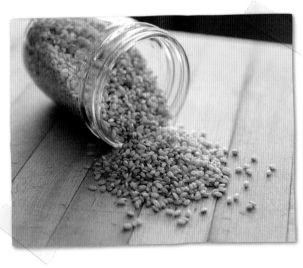

Russ, 58–59
Sally, 75, 119, 130
Sheldon, 96–97
Tebben, 150–151
herbs shopping list, 218
hidden food allergies/sensitivities, 46–50
honey substitutes, 195
hormone-based contraceptives, 78
hotels, cooking in, 146
hot flashes, 81
human welfare, 61–62
hummus, 157
hummus substitutes, 121
hypertension, 28, 29, 51, 88, 96–97

i

ice cream, 125, 126, 156, 196
iron, 73
irritability, 211
irritable bowel syndrome, 25, 41

j

Jane, 171
Jeremy (testimonial), 184–186
juices, weight and, 210
justifications, 110–111

k

Kelly, 71, 84, 85
kelp, 195
Kessler, David A., 160
KFC, 145
kidney disease, 82
kids' parties, 170
Kim (testimonial), 190–192
kitchen tools, 117, 141

l

leading by example, 181–192
    by feeding others plant-based foods, 187–189
    tailoring your message in, 183, 187
    through social media, 190–192
legumes, 46, 74.
    see also beans; lentils

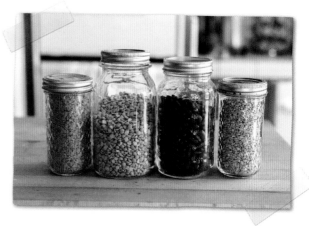

lentils, 108
lentil alternatives, 197–198
Lewis, Carl, 95
liquid smoke, 195
Lisle, Douglas J., 23, 162

m

Mackey, Bill, 100
"magic foods," 52
male pattern baldness, 86
maple syrup, 156, 195
    in baking, 203
margarines, 199
margarine substitutes, 201
mayonnaise substitutes, 157, 160, 195
McDougall, John, 32, 42, 49–50, 71, 75, 80,
    141, 178, 210
meal bars, 126
meal plans, 110, 117, 127–129.
    see also 7-Day Meal Plan

meats, 103
meats substitutes, 124–125, 195
Mediterranean diet myth, 33
men, 81–83, 86
   erectile dysfunction, 83
   male pattern baldness, 86
   prostate problems, 83
   resources for, 254
menopause, 80–81
menstruation, 80
message, tailoring, 183, 187
Michaela (Jeremy's wife), 184–186
Michelle (changes in kids
   testimonial), 88–89
Michelle (eating disorder testimonial), 163–164
migraines, 14, 25, 41
milk, asthma and, 46. *see also* dairy foods
milk protein, 154
milk substitutes, 107–108, 111, 124, 195, 205
minerals, 33–35, 73–74
minimalist meals, 127–129

miso, 195, 199
   chickpea, 196, 220
mixed-diet dinner parties, 171
mixed households, 175–178
moderation, 110–111
mood swings, 46

n

nasal congestion, 46
natural contraception, 80
negativity from others, 162, 165–166
networking, 109–110
Nixon, Scott (author's husband), 15–18
   (testimonial), 118, 122, 175–176
nondairy foods shopping list, 215
   nondairy milks, 112, 124, 196
   transitioning to, 107
non–hormone-based contraceptives, 78–79
nut butters, weight and, 210
nutrition, 23–36
   dairy myth, 24–25
   fatty acids (or fish oil) myth, 32
   "good fat" myth, 31–32
   grass-fed myth, 27, 30
   Mediterranean diet myth, 33
   oil myth, 31
   plant-based food pyramid, 36
   during pregnancy and breast-feeding, 71–75
   protein myth, 25–27, 30
   soy myth, 30–31
   vitamin and minerals deficiencies
   myth, 33–35
   vitamin B_{12} myth, 34
nutritional yeast, 195
nuts, 23, 108

o

oat flour, 203
obesity, 25, 40, 41, 45, 50–55
objections to plant-based lifestyle, 110–113,
   117–120

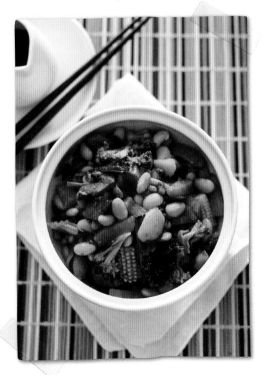

oil myth, 31
oils
    eliminating, 103
    energy density of, 53
    plant-based substitutes for, 201
    and taste buds, 161–162
    and weight gain/stalled weight loss, 210
omega-3s, 32, 73
oral allergy syndrome, 44–45
osteoporosis, 42
ovarian cysts, 75

p

pantry items shopping list, 217
parenting resources, 254–255
parties, 170, 189
people-pleasing, 173
pets, 99, 149

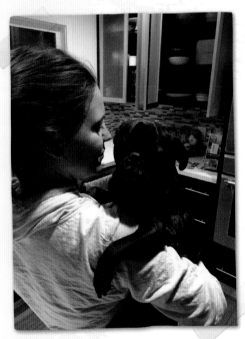

picky eaters, 113, 117
plant-based commercial substitutes, 120–122
plant-based diet, 19–36
    benefits of (*see* benefits of plant-based diet)
    challenges of (*see* challenges of plant-based lifestyle)
    cost of, 111–112, 116–117
    defined, 20
    food pyramid for, 36
    getting started with (*see* starting a plant-based lifestyle)
    global impact of, 55–62
    nutrition in, 23–35
    objections to, 110–113, 117–120
    results of (*see* results of plant-based eating)
    transitioning to (*see* transition to plant-based lifestyle)
    vegan diet vs., 21–23
plant-based food pyramid, 36
politics of food, 23–24, 256
pollution, 60
polycystic ovary syndrome (PCOS), 75–77
potatoes, 108
    buying, 116
    in elimination diet, 71
    land use for, 56
    in minimalist meals, 127–129
    protein in, 26
    and tiredness, 211
    as tofu substitute, 197
    in transition meals, 107, 108
potlucks, hosting, 189
pregnancy, 71–75, 255–256
pressure cookers, 141, 146
processed foods, 14, 103, 162
produce shopping list, 215, 217
prostate problems, 83
protein(s)
    daily need for, 26
    and meat as manly, 81–82
    milk, 154
    myth about, 25–27, 30
    and oral allergy syndrome, 44–45
    during pregnancy and breast-feeding, 72
psoriasis, 41

r

rain forest destruction, 60–61
Ras el hanout, 232
raw sugar, 204
recipes, 219–245
    adapting, 194–195, 199–200
    condiments, broths, and sauces, 237–245
    one-pot, 221–236
religion, resources on, 256
restaurant chains, 134, 145
restaurant meals. *see* eating out; traveling

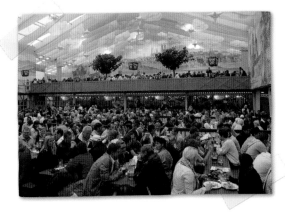

results of plant-based eating, 66–99
    for athletes, 92–97
    on bodily functions, 68–70
    for children, 86–91
    on food sensitivities and allergies, 70–71
    for men, 81–83, 86
    for pets, 99
    for women, 71–81
Robin (testimonial), 114–115, 130
Rusas, Maura Gonzales, 62
Russ (testimonial), 58–59

S

Sally (testimonial), 75, 119, 130
salt, 103, 155, 157, 161–162, 210
Schinner, Miyoko, 157
school lunches, 90

Scott, Dave, 95
seafood, 195, 196
seasonal allergies, 43–45
seaweed, 195
seeds, 23, 74, 108, 197, 210.
    see also plant-based diet
seitan, 195, 198
"selfish," being, 175
Seneca, 213
Servan-Schreiber, David, 119
7-Day Meal Plan, 110, 207
    cost of foods for, 112
    energy density basis of, 54
    fruit as sweetener in, 156
    as gluten-free, 198
    as soy- and nut-free, 197
    and tiredness, 211
sexual virility, 83
Shay, Lenore (author's mother), 102–106
    (testimonial), 188
Shay, Richard (author's father), 102–106
    (testimonial), 112, 160, 170–171, 188
Sheldon (testimonial), 96–97
shopping list, 215, 217–218
shopping on a budget, 116–117
shortening substitutes, 201
sinus congestion, 25
skin issues, 46
snacks
    available options for, 108
    for children, 91
    commercial substitutes for, 121–122
    vegan snack bars, 126
social situations, 167–173
    dinner invitations, 168–169
    "don't worry about me" approach to, 167–168
    kids' parties, 170
    politely declining food, 170–173
    standing your ground, 173
    weddings and catered events, 169
soy
    alternatives to, 196–197
    and asthma, 46
    and flatulence, 68–69

in minimalist meals, 128
  myth about, 30–31
spelt flour, 203
Standard American Diet, 40, 41
standing your ground, 173
staple foods, 116

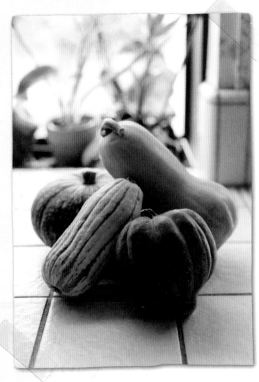

starting a plant-based lifestyle, 214–218
  by making a commitment, 214
  shopping list for, 215, 217–218
Stepaniak, Jo, 157
store brands, 122
strokes, 25, 42, 51, 79, 82
substitutions
  in baking, 199–201
  commercial (*see* commercial substitutes)
  for dairy and cheese, 157
  for fats, 157, 160
  for favorite foods, 112
  and food allergies, 196–199
  gluten-free, 218

for milk, 107–108
in recipes, 194–195
for salt, 157
soy-free, 218
for sugar, 156
vegan, 109, 122–126
sucanat, 156, 204
sugar
  addiction to, 154, 155
  in baking, 199
  baking substitutes for, 203–204
  breaking addiction to, 156
  eliminating, 103
  energy density of, 53
  as "magic food," 52
  and taste buds, 161–162
  and weight, 210
sunflower seed butter, 197
supermarkets, 144
supplements, 34, 69, 73, 74, 111
sweeteners, 156
sweetener substitutes, 203–204

t

tailoring your message, 183, 187
tamari, 198
taste buds, 161–162
Tebben (testimonial), 82, 150–151
tempeh, 69, 128, 195, 196
temptation, avoiding, 174–175
textured vegetable protein, 195
tiredness, 211. *see also* fatigue
tofu, 69, 195
tofu alternatives, 196
transition to plant-based lifestyle, 101–130
  on a budget, 116–117
  common objections to, 110–113, 117–120
  minimalist meals in, 127–129
  plant-based commercial
  substitutes, 120–122
  in small steps, 103
  stages of grief with, 113
  tips for, 107–10

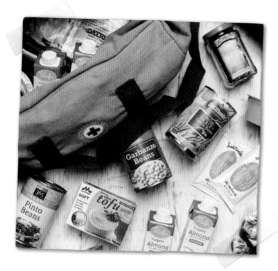

travel emergency kit, vegan, 149
traveling, 140–149
   camping and backpacking, 146–148
   grilling, 148
   hotel and dorm cooking, 146
   plant-based foods for, 141–144
   roadside restaurant chains, 145
   supermarkets and fruit stands, 144
   vegan travel emergency kit, 149
   websites and apps, 145
tree nuts, 196
turbinado sugar, 204

U

uterine fibroids, 75

V

veganism, 16–17
   and asthma incidence, 46
   plant-based diet vs., 21–23
   and weight loss, 55
vegan substitute foods, 122–126
vegan travel emergency kit, 149
vegan travel foods, 143–144

vegetarianism, 14
   and allergies, 43
   and asthma incidence, 43, 46
   plant-based diet vs., 20
   veg-friendly cuisines, 134–136
   and weight loss, 55
vitamin B$_{12}$, 34, 74
vitamin D, during pregnancy, 75
vitamins, 33–35, 73–75

W

water resources, 56–57
weddings, 169
weight loss, 15–18, 50–55
   stalled, 210–211
wheat
   as allergen, 196
   alternatives to, 198
white chocolate, 205
whole grains, 23, 74, 108. *see also* plant-based diet
whole-wheat flours, 202–203
willpower, 118
women, 71–81
   contraception, 78–80
   fertility, 75–78
   menopause, 80–81
   menstruation, 80
   pregnancy and breast-feeding nutrition, 71–75
world hunger, 56
wraps, substitutes for, 121

Y

yogurt, 196. *see also* dairy foods
yogurt substitutes, 124

Z

zinc, 74

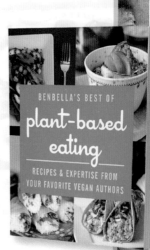
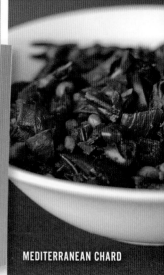
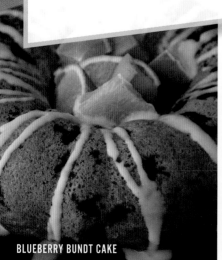
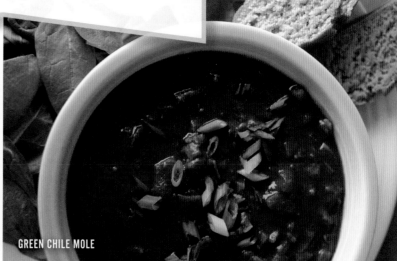
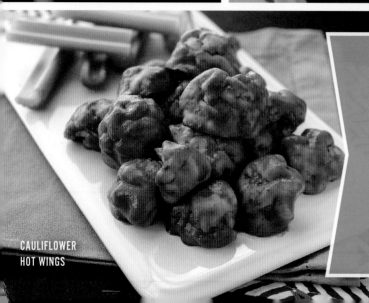